After you finish this book,
a

NO

will be your most probable reply to doctors, who invariably offer you chemotherapy, radiotherapy, surgery, vaccination and the so-called life saving drugs to prevent, control or cure any of your diagnosed medical conditions.

Cancer | Vaccination | Heart Disease | Thyroid

| Diabetes | Genetic disorder | Tuberculosis | HIV-AIDS | COVID19 |

| Hypertension | Surgery | Kidney failure | Paralysis | Auto immune disease |

1 Question that can save your life

By
Dr. Biswaroop Roy Chowdhury

Asthma | Pneumonia | Infertility | Ulcer | IBS

DIAMOND BOOKS

BROUGHT TO YOU BY
Indo-Vietnam Medical Board

India Office:
C/o India Book of Records
B-121, 2nd Floor, Greenfields,
Faridabad -12003 (Haryana), India
Ph. :+91-9312286540

Vietnam Office:
C/o Vietnam Book of Records
148 Hong Ha Street
9 Award, Phu Nhuan District,
Ho Chi Minh City, Vietnam
- Hotline: (+84) 903710505

Malaysia Office:
C/o Biswaroop International Healing & Research
PT 573, Lot 15077 Jalan Tuanku Munawir,
70000 Negeri Sembilan, Malaysia
Tel :+6012-2116089

Switzerland Office:
C/o Nigel Kingsley
Kraftwerkstr. 95, ch-5465, Mellikon, Switzerland
Tel : 0041 79 222 2323

FOLLOW ME
Video Channel: www.coronakaal.tv
Email: biswaroop@biswaroop.com
Website: www.biswaroop.com

Research: Rachna Sharma

Patient Coordination: Kalpana Bourai, Dr, Sanju Khari

Proof Reading: Sonum Garg

Graphics Designer: Shankar Singh Koranga

Published By:
Diamond Pocket Books
X-30, OKhla Industrial Area, New Delhi-110020
Tel.: 011-40712200
Email:sales@dpb.in Website:www.diamondbook.in

DEDICATION

Dedicated to my angel daughter Ivy,

loving wife Neerja

&

caring parents

Shri Bikash Roy Chowdhury

Shrimati Lila Roy Chowdhury

CONTENTS

SECTION -I

One question
that can save your life
(Evidences v/s Expectation)

One question that can save your life

Had Mr. George Washington questioned his doctors, he would have increased his lifespan to a great extent.

It was December 14, 1799 when the first President of America Mr. George Washington got fever and was caught in the grip of Flu. When he went to the hospital for treatment (the popular method of treatment at that time was bloodletting i.e., to let the blood flow out of the body), his blood was let out of the body. That is, whenever a patient came to the hospital with fever, a cut was made with a blade and the blood was let to flow out of the body. It was considered that by letting the blood flow out, the fever would be cured.

As per the treatment, the blood was let out of George Washington's body but the fever remained as it was and by evening or so, almost half the amount of blood was removed from his body and he died. The next day, a press release was issued by the doctors saying that we regret Mr. George Washington came to our hospital for treatment and we started letting the blood out from his body till it was reduced to half, even then we could not save him.

If we keep in mind today's evidence, it appears that Mr. Washington passed away not due to fever but due to excessive loss of blood from the body.

Earlier a science journalist named Mr. William Cobbett had collected all the evidences and showed it to the world that this method of letting the blood flow out of the body to cure fever was leading to more deaths in comparison to those people who were not taking any treatment for fever. But Mr. George Washington ignored the evidence and relied on the popular method rather than paying attention to what the evidence was pointing towards.

Those doctors, whose livelihood depended on this method of letting the blood flow out of the body, filed a case against Mr. William Cobbett. He lost the case, got bankrupt and was even exiled. As a result, such treatment continued for the next 200 years. The state of medical science that persisted in those days, exists even today.

Let us take a simple medical condition say, Diabetes. If you want to save your life, you must ask the doctor one question 'Do you have any evidence that by taking this particular medicine for Diabetes, my lifespan will increase or my quality of life will improve?' Shockingly, there is no evidence to prove that by taking any medicine for Diabetes, the lifespan would increase or the quality of life would improve.

On the contrary, there are major trials like ACCORD trial, VADTS trial & UKPDS trial, which conclusively reveal that these medicines decrease the lifespan and worsen the quality of life in comparison to not consuming any medicine.

All the medicines, whether for Blood Sugar or Blood Pressure, just provide a number – a number that you may fancy (my Blood Sugar should be this and Blood Pressure should be that) at the cost of making you more sick; even at the cost of killing you.

Let us say there are two people. Both of them have the same disease (Blood Sugar or Blood Pressure) to the same degree; one decides to follow all the medicines prescribed by the doctor and the other could not take medicines due to some reason. After a few years, it was observed that the person, who had consumed the medicines prescribed by the doctor, had much higher mortality rate in comparison to the one who did not take the medicines (though he was sick, too).

Whatever I have explained for Diabetes or Hypertension holds true for Cancer as well. A patient suffering from Cancer too must question the doctor, "On your advice, I am undergoing Chemotherapy or surgery or radiation, but do you have any evidence to show that by doing so, my lifespan will increase or my quality of life will improve?" Shockingly, there is no evidence to prove that your lifespan will increase or your quality of life will improve by these popular treatments. On the contrary, there are evidences to show that your lifespan will decrease and your quality of life will deteriorate.

Following are the evidences of the evaluation of the effectiveness of major medical interventions in question & answer format:

Q1) Is there any evidence that by undergoing the diagnosis for Cancer (biopsy/mammography etc.) so as to decide the treatment protocol, will my lifespan increase or my quality of life improve in comparison to not undergoing the diagnosis at all ?

Ans: There is no evidence that the diagnosis for Cancer, will in anyway, help you to live a longer life or improve the quality of life; however it is well established that the biopsies suppress the immune system and promote Cancer metastasis.[71-75]

Similarly, in the case of mammography, the breast is tightly and often painfully[76] compressed between two imaging plates. If Cancer is present in the breast, the compression can result in metastasis.[77]

On the contrary, avoiding repeated mammography may lead to at least 22% chances of spontaneous regression.

In other words, by simply avoiding the repeated dose of ionizing radiation administered during mammography, the body is given a chance to heal on its own and often it does[78].

Q2) Is there any evidence that reducing the fever by taking antipyretic drugs (Paracetamol etc.) helps in curing the illness faster or increasing the lifespan or improving the quality of life in comparison to not taking any medicine for fever control?

Ans: There is no evidence in medical literature to prove that taking antipyretic medicines to reduce fever helps in any way other than providing temporary symptomatic comfort. However, there are evidences suggesting that antipyretics may lead to reduced survival and increased duration of suffering.[79]

Q3) Is there any evidence that by controlling blood sugar with medication can help in improving the quality of life and increasing the lifespan in comparison to not taking any medicine?

Ans: There is no large-scale evidence to support consumption of medicines for Diabetes. However, there is a clear-cut evidence that by consuming medicines to control the blood sugar may increase the rate of mortality by 22%.[80]

Q4) Is there any evidence that controlling blood pressure with medication can help in improving the quality of life and increasing the lifespan in comparison to not taking any medicine?

Ans: There is no evidence to support that consuming blood pressure medicines can improve the quality of a person's life or increase his lifespan. However, there is clear cut evidence to show that by consuming medicines to control blood pressure may increase the rate of mortality[81].

Q5) Is there any evidence that by taking the recommended vaccine will help in increasing the lifespan or improving the quality of life of a person in comparison to not taking any vaccine?

Ans: There is no evidence in medical literature to prove that getting vaccinated will help one live a longer life or improve the quality of life. However, there are evidences to prove the opposite.[82,83,84]

Q6) Is there any evidence to prove that by taking the treatment in accordance with the current WHO protocol (Remdesivir, hydroxychloroquine, antibiotics, antipyretics etc.) will help in faster recovery of COVID-19 patients or increase their chances of survival?

Ans: There is no evidence to prove that the WHO protocol will be of any help to the COVID-19 patients. However the SOLIDARITY trial[85] of WHO concludes: about 12% death rate and over 80% of the patients with long term side effects .

On the other hand, more than 50,000 COVID-19 /ILI patients were treated with the 3-Step Flu Diet with zero death and zero side effects with 95% of them having recovered in 3 days and 100% of them in 14 days.[86]

Q7) Is there any evidence to show that using normal saline intravenously can help a patient in recovering faster or improving his chances of recovery?

Ans: There is no evidence to support that the widespread use of normal saline intravenously will enable a patient to recover faster or improve his chances of recovery whereas there is evidence to show that it causes kidney damage /failure[87].

Q8) Is there any evidence to show that bypass surgery & angioplasty can help a patient with blocked arteries live a longer life or improve his quality of life in comparison to not undergoing any such procedures ?

Ans: There is no evidence to prove that bypass surgery / angioplasty can help a person to improve his quality of life or increase his lifespan. However there are evidences to prove the other way round.[88-90]

Besides, we must remember that bypass surgeries come with potential complications like impotency,[91] brain damage and organ dysfunction[92].

Q9) Is there any evidence to prove that Chemotherapy can help a Cancer patient to live longer or improve his quality of life in comparison to not undergoing Chemotherapy ?

Ans: There are no evidences to prove that Chemotherapy helps a Cancer patient to improve his quality of life or increase his life span. On the contrary, there are sufficient evidences to prove otherwise.[93-96]

Here the point to understand is the shrinking of the initial tumor mass, chemotherapy deceives the doctors into thinking that the patients are benefitting from the treatment, when in reality, the growth and spread of Cancer gets accelerated by it.

Q10) Is there any evidence to prove that Radiotherapy can help a Cancer patient to live longer or improve his quality of life in comparison to not taking it ?

Ans : There are no evidences to prove that Radiotherapy can help a Cancer patient improve his quality of life or to increase his life span. On the contrary, there are sufficient evidences to prove otherwise.[97-100]

Q11) Is there any evidence to show that by eliminating the tumour with surgery can help a patient live a longer life or improve his quality of life in comparison to not undergoing surgery for eliminating tumour ?

Ans: Recent evidences show that cutting out a tumour either provides no benefit to the patients[101,102] or increases the mortality.[103-105]

The more the body is cut, the worse is the outcome.

Cancer metastasis is the primary cause of most Cancer deaths[106-108] and yes, the public remains unaware that surgical removal of tumour causes Cancer metastasis [109-116].

Q12) Why are Chemotherapy, radiation and surgery the most popular and widespread treatment protocols all over the world, even though there is no evidence of benefit?

Ans: If you go through the poster given in this book, you will know that Chemotherapy / Surgery causes damage to all the organs of the body. If a patient undergoes chemotherapy and later suffers a heart attack and dies within a week/month/year, in such a case, the cause of death is deemed to be the heart attack rather than a cancer death as a result of the side effects of the anti-cancer treatments.

Evidence of this can be seen in studies reporting decreased rate of cancer deaths, while simultaneously increasing number of non-cancer deaths following Radiotherapy treatment.[117-119]

Similarly, by examining non-cancer deaths of 470,000 cancer patients, as published in the journal of the National Cancer Institute, the study found out that 27% of the patients who were reported dead for reasons, other than cancer, had died within a year after diagnosis suggesting that they were probably killed by the treatment procedures.[120]

Q13) Is there any evidence that the knee Arthroscopy (for Arthritis) can help in improving the quality of life?

Ans: In a placebo controlled (sham surgery) study over two years, no difference has been found between the groups in terms of knee pain or function.[121]

Q14) Is there any evidence that hysterectomy can improve the quality of life or increase the lifespan in comparison to not undergoing it?

Ans: The unintended consequences of removing women's ovaries leads to complications like heart disease, stroke, Parkinson's disease, dementia and osteoporosis.

There is also evidence to show that by removing the ovaries (while decreasing your chances of dying from ovarian cancer) increases your overall chances of dying,[122]

Q15) Is there any evidence to prove that antibiotics can help a patient of respiratory illness recover faster in comparison to not consuming them at all?

Ans: There is no evidence to support that antibiotics treat flu or respiratory diseases; however, there are evidences against it.[123]

Q16) Is it recommended to go for general preventive health check- ups?

Ans: According to Cochrane Collaboration, who included 17 randomized controlled trials, came to the conclusion that systematic offers of health check-ups are unlikely to benefit and may lead to unnecessary tests and treatment.

Then, what should we do? Should we simply sit down without doing anything? No! You just have to find out the evidence-based treatment? Remember, whether it is a lifestyle disease or infectious disease or even a genetic disorder, nature has umpteen ways to cure you of your illness; which in turn can increase your life span and improve the quality of your life.

In order to make you understand, let me give you an example with evidence-Congenital heart disease or hole in the heart.

What is hole in the heart (Atrial Septal defect)?

Normally, the right side of the heart pumps oxygen- rich blood to the body. When a person has a hole in the heart (ASD), blood from the left & right sides mix and cause various health issues.

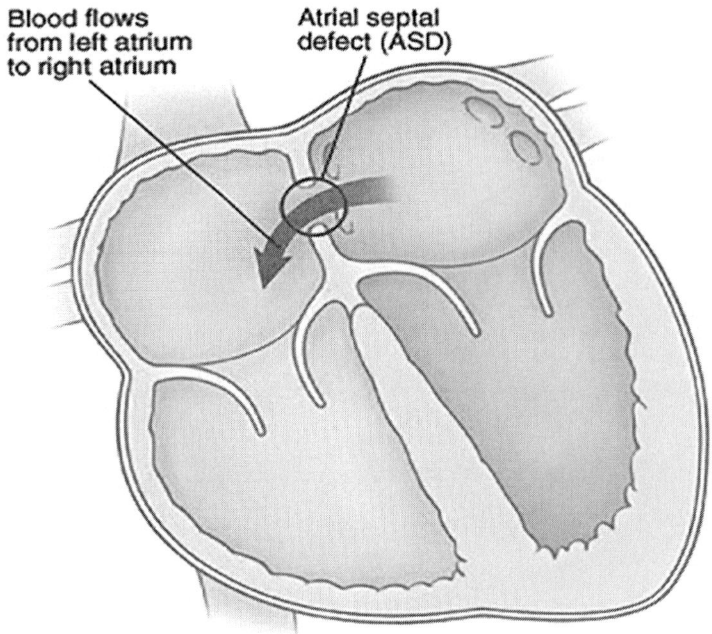

Atrial Septal Defect

Sometimes, this disorder is diagnosed towards the later part of the life while remaining symptom free for a major part of the life.

If you want to go through the case study of one such person then you can go to the link www.coronakaal.tv/asd and watch the video of Mr. Subash Chand Sharma.

When the doctors denied any hope of survival,they decided to follow the DIP diet and within a few days of following the DIP diet, the size of the hole got reduced; the oxygen cylinder had to be removed and he, once again, resumed his work.

This seems impossible but he made it possible. I have already put in all the evidences on the given link www.biswaroop.com/evidences

Now imagine a child born with not one but four defects in the heart namely:

1. Hole in the heart
2. Pulmonary stenosis (narrowing of the pulmonary valve leading to lack of blood flow to the lungs)

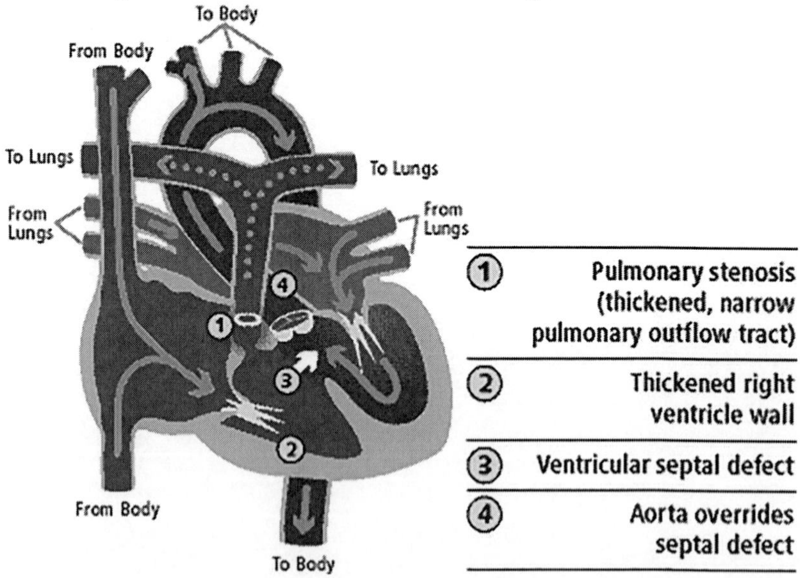

3. Right ventricular hypertrophy (thickening of the walls of right ventricle)
4. Overriding aorta (causing oxygen- poor blood flow to aorta instead of pulmonary artery)

This happens in the rarest of rare cases. This is called Tetralogy of Fallot. Such a child is incurable according to conventional science. But if such children take DIP diet; they can recover in a few months. I am giving you evidence of one such child in this video **www.coronakaal.tv/onequestion**

Script of video testimonial as narrated by our diabetes educator 'Sripad Baidya'

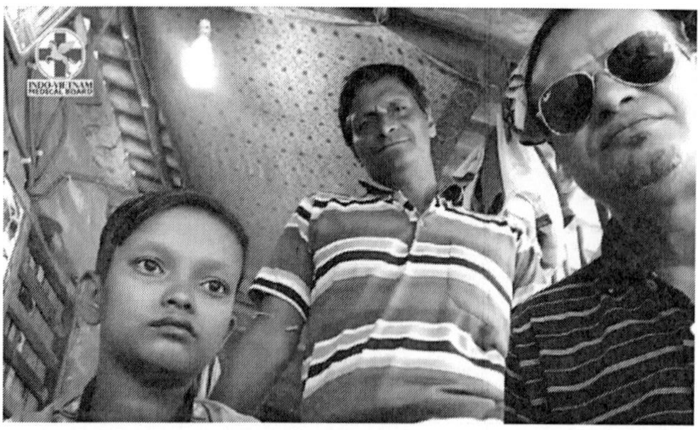

Joy Baidya , father of Joy Baidya & Sripad Baidya (Diabetes Educator)

Greetings! I am Sripad Baidya , Indo -Vietnam Board Diabetes Educator. The example of the result of standard DIP diet 3rd gear diet and 4th gear diet-which is a popular diet- is in front of me-Joy Baidya. I came to a remote village of Sunderban area in West Bengal- district 24 Parganas North, Block, panchayat-Govindgadi.

I came to this village and gave the diet prescribed by Dr. Biswaroop Roy Chowdhury to Joy (Joy's father is also present). The child was born in 2007 with a heart disease but the disease was not diagnosed till 2019. In March 2020, he had a severe problem for which he was admitted to PG hospital.

In the diagnosis, after admission, he was referred to Rabindranath Tagore hospital for operation. The diagnosis was referred to as TOF (Tetrology of Fallot)

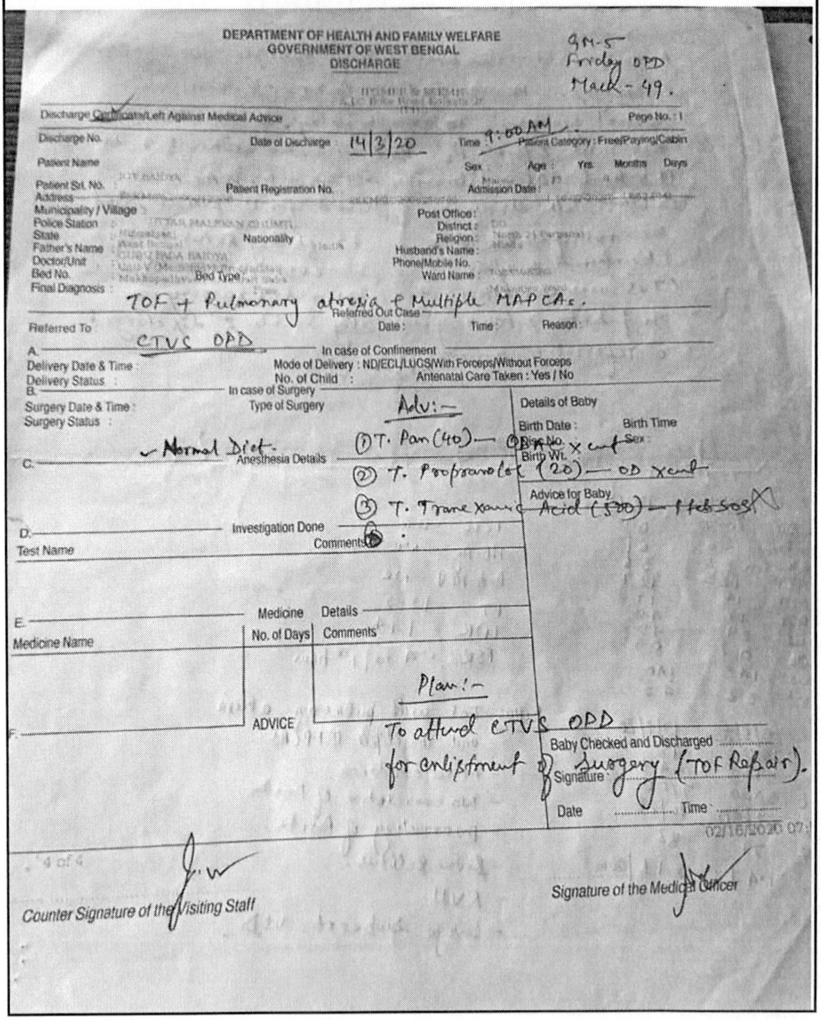

DEPARTMENT OF HEALTH AND FAMILY WELFARE
GOVERNMENT OF WEST BENGAL
DISCHARGE

Discharge Certificate/Left Against Medical Advice — Page No. : 1

Discharge No. — Date of Discharge: 14/3/20 — Time: 9:00 AM — Patient Category: Free/Paying/Cabin

Patient Name — Sex — Age: Yrs Months Days

Patient Srl. No. — Patient Registration No. — Admission Date:

Address

Municipality / Village — Post Office:

Police Station — District:

State — Nationality — Religion:

Father's Name — Husband's Name:

Doctor/Unit — Phone/Mobile No.

Bed No. — Bed Type — Ward Name

Final Diagnosis: TOF + Pulmonary atresia c̄ Multiple MAPCAs.

Referred To: CTVS OPD — Referred Out Case — Date: — Time: — Reason:

A. In case of Confinement
Delivery Date & Time: — Mode of Delivery: ND/ECL/LUCS/With Forceps/Without Forceps
Delivery Status: — No. of Child: — Antenatal Care Taken: Yes / No

B. In case of Surgery
Surgery Date & Time: — Type of Surgery — Details of Baby
Surgery Status: — Birth Date: — Birth Time

C. Normal Diet. — Anesthesia Details

Adv:–
① T. Pan (40) — OD BF × cont
② T. Propranolol (20) — OD × cont
③ T. Tranexamic Acid (500) — 1 tab SOS

D. Investigation Done
Test Name — Comments

E. Medicine Details
Medicine Name — No. of Days — Comments

F. ADVICE
Plan:–
To attend CTVS OPD for enlistment of Surgery (TOF Repair).

Baby Checked and Discharged
Signature
Date — Time

Counter Signature of the Visiting Staff — Signature of the Medical Officer

It is a rare disease occurring in a few children. The poor family of Joy spent whatever lifetime savings they had for the life of this 13-year old child. The child used to bleed every month starting from 2007; he was losing weight and his growth was inhibited. There was blackness/bluishness (Cyanosis) in his body due to the disease as the pure blood and impure blood was mixing up.

The family could not get Joy operated due to lockdown imposed by the government in the month of March. How successful would it have been is an entirely different question? He could not be admitted since the doctors refused surgery at that time. Since they did not have money to stay there, they returned to the village. They have a small house in the village and they live in abject poverty as you can see.

These people contacted us and we mailed all the details to Indo-Vietnam Medical Board Dr. Biswaroop Roy Chowdhury who prescribed 4th gear diet to be given to the child. The effect started to be seen. For the last 9-10 months, he has no problem; he has started gaining weight; his breathing problem has vanished; and a positive change can be seen on his face; his blood vomiting has also stopped completely.

This family now has immense faith on this diet. With this trust, the child's father would say a few words:

This child was born in 2007 and after the birth, the child had heart problem. We went to several doctors at several places and whatever medicines they prescribed, we gave to the child but they had no effect. In March 2020, he was admitted to PG. But due to lockdown, they did not perform operation. We are poor people; what would we eat there; we had no money so we returned to our village. With the diet he was given (which continues even now), the child is better now. He does not puke out blood from the mouth and his face has also changed. The child is right here. He has no problem. In all, there is belief on this system; there is faith and, in the days to come, he wants to continue with the system.

After reading the story of Joy, you must have realized that there are simple ways to cure any kind of disease; and that one of the ways is called 'The DIP Diet'. I have given you enough evidences in the following sections of this book but if you need more, then you can go to the link www.coronakaal.tv and under 'testimonials' section, you can watch thousands of evidences containing video testimonials.

You may have any disease whether diabetes, heart disease, kidney failure, thyroid, arthritis or infectious disease like COVID-19 or HIV AIDS- you can cure them through DIP diet.

If you wish to learn, how DIP diet can cure a particular disease, you can do so absolutely free of cost. All you have to do is to go to the link 'www.coronakaal.tv' and click on 'CURE ME' section.

This section has a collection of videos which explain the use of DIP diet for treating various kinds of diseases. Through these self-explanatory videos you can easily undergo treatment at home (without anyone's help) by following the diet plan and reverse your sickness no matter what that is, in just a few days.

But there will be some people who wish to be treated under our supervision; they can click on www.biswaroop.com/wise (W.I.S.E stands for Wellness and Inflammatory Syndrome Experts). We have around 500 experts and you have been recently introduced to one expert named Sripad Baidya, who cured Joy.

These 500 experts will guide you (through video conferencing) on how DIP diet is to be taken based on the disease and also provide you with a three-week diet protocol. For this, the first step is to fill up the form: www.biswaroop.com/wise.

The second step is to deposit Rs 500 in the account of that expert. Remember, that the W.I.S.E form can be filled only by those who suffer from just one disease- like Diabetes or Hypertension or Thyroid or Tuberculosis and the disease should be in the initial stages or the patient should have a medical history of less than 5 years. Given below is the list of diseases covered under W.I.S.E.

- High Blood Pressure
- High Cholesterol
- Constipation
- Urinary Tract Infection
- Low Blood Pressure
- Angina
- Piles
- Ulcer
- Fatty Liver
- Hepatitis
- Anemia
- Obesity
- Thyroid
- Low Body Weight
- Enlarged Prostate
- Diabetes Type 2
- Pre-Menstrual Syndrome / Painful Periods /
- Periods With Excessive Bleeding / Pcod
- Cataract
- Kidney Stone
- Weak Immunity
- Insomnia
- Liver Cirrhosis
- Impotency
- Sinusitis
- Asthma
- Bronchitis
- Eczema
- Back Pain
- Migraine
- Depression
- Varicose Veins
- Parkinson
- Alzheimer
- Dementia
- Psoriasis
- Joint Pain
- Sciatica
- Spondylosis
- Infertility
- Acidity
- Gas
- Ibs

Still, there may be a few people who are suffering from multiple medical conditions and complications; like kidney failure and hence on dialysis; has heart disease and is on medication for diabetes; is sick for the last 20/30 years- for such complicated cases, you can go to the link www.biswaroop.com/vopd and fill up the form. Such cases are personally handled by me and my core team. For such cases, first fill up the Virtual OPD/ VOPD form. After reviewing the form, we will get in touch with you. Fee for personal consultation through VOPD is Rs 21,000. The profile of that patient will be personally viewed by me and I will tell you how you should include DIP diet in your life, so that you gradually come out of the trap of medicines and get rid of diseases; increase your life span and improve the quality of your life.

In the end, I would again emphasize that whenever you choose a particular treatment, before starting the treatment, you must question the doctor that; "if I consume these medicines or follow your treatment, will it increase my lifespan and improve the quality of my life in comparison to avoiding any treatment altogether"? If he is able to provide some evidence, only then proceed for that treatment.

In the following sections (II, III and IV) of this book I have included some of the successful case studies of my patients as an evidence of effectiveness of the DIP Diet. So, read on...

REFERENCES

To access the references, go to the link **www.biswaroop.com/onequestion**

SECTION -II

Hiding the truth to save Diabetes Industry (Diabetes type 1 reversal case study - Journal of the Science of Healing Outcomes)

Hiding the truth to save Diabetes industry

For the first time in the history of medical science, a Diabetic Type 1 patient after remaining Insulin dependent (60 units per day) for more than seven years, could reverse diabetes and her dependency on Insulin just by following the DIP Diet.

This case study got published in the 50th issue (Jan 2021) of 'Journal of the Science of Healing Outcomes'

This journal is highly reputed because of the distinguished editorial team which includes Padam Bhushn Dr. B.M Hegde (Editor In-charge), Brian Josephson (Nobel Laureate) and Richard Smith (former Editor of British Medical Journal) & Vice Chancellors of Universites.

However, it would be no surprise if this case study is being censored from getting published in main stream media, as it may lead to extinction of the very Diabetes/Drug/Insulin Industry, which funds the mainstream media.

In the next few pages find the case study copied as it is from the 'Journal of the Science of Healing Outcomes'.

Biswroop Roy Chowdhury

Reversal of Type 1 Diabetes Using Plant Based Diet: A Case Study

Abstract

Type 1 diabetes (T1D) is an autoimmune disease characterized by hyperglycemia, the inability to produce insulin due to self destruction of beta cells in the pancreas. The disorder of type 1 diabetes causes irreversible damages like retinopathy, nephropathy, neuropathy, foot complications, high blood pressure, and puts patients on a life sentence with insulin. The common perception in medical science is that sugar levels cannot be normalized without the help of medication. However, in the present study we examined a suspected type 1 diabetic patient by putting her on a diet plan with regular follow ups and studied all diabetes-related biochemical parameters. We were successfully able to eliminate her medication and insulin dependency.

Diabetes is one of the most common metabolic disorders associated with many life threatening complications which make the life of a diabetic person worse. Diabetes is of two types-type 1 diabetes (T1D) and type 2 diabetes (T2D). T2D is the more common type of diabetes worldwide (90-95%), marked by an increased blood sugar level, frequent urination and weight loss. The other is T1D or gestational diabetes (5-10%). In T2D, impaired receptors do not respond to insulin, eventually leading to insulin resistance while in T1D, there is a deficiency of insulin[1] . Out of all diabetes cases 1-2% cases are Maturity Onset Diabetes of the Young[2] (MODY).

According to a recent estimate of International Diabetes Federation, South East Asia region, in 2017 there were 72,946,400 diabetic cases in

India, 425 million cases in the world and 82 million in South East Asia region, which is likely to go up to 151 million by 2045[3] . According to an estimate drawn in 2015, India has about 97,700 children with type 1 diabetes mellitus (T1DM or T1D)4 .

Although T1D is not as prevalent as T2D, it shows a trend of 3–5% increase every year. India itself records three new cases of T1DM/100,000 children in the age group of 0–14 years. Prevalence data of three regions shows 17.93 cases/100,000 children in Karnataka, 3.2 cases/100,000 children in Chennai and 10.2 cases/100,000 children in Karnal (Haryana) of T1D. It is a juvenile onset disorder which is characterized by pancreatic dysfunction due to autoimmune reaction of the body where beta cells continuously get destroyed, eventually leading to insulin deficiency[6] .

One highly sensitive method of C-peptide determination has shown that beta cells can be detected even up to 40 years after the clinical onset of the disease. These findings help patients in advanced stage, for example, it helps patients whose β-cell function was thought to have long ceased in getting benefit from interventions to preserve β-cell function or to prevent complications[7] . Alot of effort has been made to regenerate beta cells in vitro by providing growth factors and by reprogramming/transdifferentiation of terminally differentiated cell types. However, none of these approaches have proved to be successful in growing beta cells in vivo due to shortage of donors. The inefficient technique of β-cell generation and the difficulty of growing β-cell in adult humans sufficiently force a patient to adhere to medication for his whole life[8] . Change in food habits plays an important role in both type 1 and type 2 diabetes by modulating or completely restoring normal glucose levels, thereby either decreasing or eliminating the need of medicine/insulin[9] .

Case presentation

Here, we present a case of a 23-year-old female, weighing 60 kg, who was diagnosed with diabetes at Fortis, Mohali on 28 December 2011. She had been on insulin (60 U/day) for eight years before coming to us. She was diagnosed with T1D at 15 years of age and came to us at 23 years. Moreover, she was on insulin from the very first day, did not show any family history and showed higher values of Hb1Ac (9.3%) which are suggestive of T1D than MODY.

Furthermore, in the absence of initial C-peptide and Glutamic Acid Decarboxylase (GAD) reports diagnosis was difficult. However, such negligence in maintaining records by the clinical practitioners should be avoided which leads to such discrepancies in diagnosis. She complained about her vision, and was diagnosed with glaucoma in both her eyes and retinal detachment in her left eye. Her eyes had been operated on thrice. She displayed a nephropathy condition as stones were also found in her kidney

She had been taking basic intervention through our video[10] for five months (August 2018-December 2018), after which, she approached us in January 2019. She was put on intensive intervention, where she was monitored for 72 hours by a six member health team in Faridabad.

Intervention

For the initial five months, she had been following the video recommended diet that included cooked food along with raw food. This diet was divided into breakfast, lunch and dinner. Breakfast included four different types of fruits which weighed equal to body weight (in kg)×10 = ...(gm). Lunch included four types of raw vegetables which weighed equal to body weight (in kg) ×5 = ... (gm) along with a normal cooked meal. Dinner was calculated the same way as lunch. In addition to this, soaked nuts and sprouts were also a part of the diet and the quantity of these also was based on the patient's body weight (kg)... (gm).

Sunshine was also an integral part of the prescribed diet. Packed and refined food, nutritional supplements, nonsteroidal anti-inflammatory drugs (NSAIDs), animal, dairy products and dinner at late hours were strictly denied.

After five months, she was recommended to follow a more restricted diet plan mainly consisting of fruits and raw vegetables. Dairy products and cooked food were completely eliminated during intensive intervention[9]. A regular monitoring of glucose (fasting and post prandial) was carried out during intervention.

Table showing biochemical parameters before and after intervention

	Date	Insulin	C-peptide	GAD	HbA1c(%)	Blood sugar in average (mg/dl)
At the time of diagnosis 2011	(28.12.11)	Mixtard 28U+22U/day Actrapid 10U/day	–	—	9.3	160*
Basic intervention (2019)	Till mid August	50 U	–	–	–	156*
	From mid Aug to Dec	25U				159*
Intensive intervention (2019)	4th Jan	0	–	–	–	195
	5th Jan	0	–	–	–	181
	6th Jan	0	–	–	–	176
At the time of writing the article		0	.93 10.02.2019	7.0 05.03.2019	7.2 18.02.2019	

GAD=gluttamic acid decarboxylase Parenthesis (-) represents the non availability of data *glucose with insulin therapy

Biochemical parameters

Before intervention

The patient had been suffering from T1D for eight years as was diagnosed in December 2011. She was prescribed Mixtard insulin 28 units before breakfast and 22 units before dinner and Actrapid 10 units before lunch. In addition to that, she was taking 1000mg of Metformin per day. Her blood sugar level varied from 156±24 mg/dl with total insulin (60 Unit) and 159±5 with 25U insulin. Her HbA1c was 9.3% (2011) and mean plasma glucose was 197 at the time of diagnosis. (Table)

Post intervention

The intervention was divided into two phases.

Basic intervention,where cooked food was offered along with raw food (August 2018-January 2019). Her dependency on insulin decreased gradually from 60U to 25U during basic intervention.

Intensive intervention, where no cooked food was given (4-6 January 2019). She was no longer dependent on insulin during intensive intervention phase. Her HBA1c was 7.2% post intervention. Her C-peptide level was .93 (.81-3.85) ng/ml, mean plasma glucose was 160 and GAD, 7 U/ml (value <30 is considered negative) after dietary intervention (Table).

Discussion

T1D has been neglected for a long time and its nationwide prevalence is not yet known. The growing number of T1D cases is a cause of concern as its treatment is difficult in comparison to that of T2D11. In this article, we show a comprehensive analysis by stating the pre and post diabetic conditions of a proband severely affected case of suspected T1D who approached us in January 2019. She was diagnosed with diabetes at the age of 18 years and from the very first day she was on insulin. She did not show any family history of diabetes and her pre intervention HbA1c reading was 9.3%, which is on the higher side. All the evidences so far define her a T1D case than any other type of diabetes.

Her higher values of HBA1c are suggestive of diabetic complications[12] which are evident by her eye and kidney problems. Her insulin dependency reduced to less than half after a basic dietary intervention, and finally, to nil after intensive intervention. Originally, when she was diagnosed as diabetic, her insulin intake was 60U (2011) per day, and it came down to 25U (2018) per day owing to dietary intervention. Presently, she is no longer dependent on insulin. Her glucose levels are also in normal range without insulin (184±9). Her GAD values are suggestive of the reversal of type 1 diabetes. She adheres to regular follow ups.

Evidences of cases of T1D due to disturbed lifestyle are increasing[13]. Dietary intervention is a great help to medical science in curbing diabetes to a large extent, without causing any side effects. The complete reversal of chronic T1D through dietary intervention is a ray of hope to many patients who are in the trap of medicines.

Acknowledgements

The author thanks Dynamic Memory Pvt. Ltd. for financial support.

References

1. Diagnosis and Classification of Diabetes Mellitus Diabetes Care Volume 37, Supplement 1, January 2014

2. Juszczak A, Pryse R, Schuman A, Owen KR. When to consider a diagnosis of MODY at the presentation of diabetes: aetiology matters for correct management. Br J Gen Pract. 2016;66(647):e457–e459.

3 . International Diabetes Federation Available from: https://www.idf.org/our-network/regions-members/southeast-asia/members/94-india.html, accessed on 29 April 2019.

4.. Kanakatte Mylariah Prasanna Kumar Incidence trends for childhood type 1 diabetes in India Indian Journal of Endocrinology and Metabolism, 2015, 19, 34-35

5. DasAK, Type 1 diabetes in India: Overall insights. Indian J Endocrinol Metab. 2015 Apr; 19 (Suppl 1): S31–S33.

6. American Diabetes Association. Classification and Diagnosis of Diabetes. Diabetes Care 2016, 39, 13-22.

7. Wang L, Lovejoy NF, Faustman DL. Persistence of prolonged C-peptide production in type 1 diabetes as measured with an ultra sensitive C-peptide assay. Diabetes Care. 2012,35:465-70.

8. Tesemma Sileshi Chala & Getnet Yimer Ali Recent advance in diabetes therapy: pancreatic beta cell regeneration approaches 2016 Volume 6, Issue 6

9. Chowdhary B R, Diabetes Reversal by Plant-Based Diet, Journal of Metabolic Syndrome, 6:4, 2017

10. Diabetes Type I, and II cure in 72 hours Available from https://www.youtube.com/watch?v=BbGWZkBl5Hg

11. Chowdhury BR (2016) For Doctors & Care Givers

12. Zoungas S, Chalmers J, Ninomiya T, Li Q, Cooper ME, Colagiuri S et al, ADVANCE Collaborative Group. Association of HbA1c levels with vascular complications and death in patients with type 2 diabetes: evidence of glycaemic thresholds. Diabetologia. 2012 Mar;55(3):636- 43.

13. Stanisław Piłaciński and Dorota A. ZozulińskaZiółkiewicz Influence of lifestyle on the course of type 1 diabetes mellitus Arch Med Sci. 2014, 10: 124–134.

SECTION -III

Effectiveness of the DIP Diet on 102 case-studies of life threatening/rare & medically incurable diseases

Watch video testimonial at www.coronakaal.tv/onequestion

1

Tongue Cancer & Thalassemia

Medical history of the patient at the time when he contacted us :

Ramesh Sachdeva, 67yrs, from New Delhi India contacted us on 3 May 2020 through Virtual OPD/VOPD

Diagnosis : TONGUE CANCER (Squamous Cell Carcinoma) detected in January 2020, Coronary artery disease since 8 years, thalassemia minor,HLA-B27 Positive cataract in both eyes, low Blood Pressure, Pre-Diabetic

Discomforts : Acidity, Constipation, Sinusitis, Mouth ulcers and sores, pain and swelling in tongue, pain in gums discomfort in eating, drinking and speaking, difficulty in breathing from nose while lying down, cough and mucus.

Medicines / Medical Intervention: Pan-D, Ganaton Total, Brilinta 90mg, Metolar XR 50, Rozucor ASP 75/20, Ativan 4mg,Dulcoflex,Gemcal, Forcan 150mg, Becosule, Ambrolite S Syrup, Antoxid, Vitamin D, Montair LC, Ensure Plus Powder, Disperzyme tab, Zerodol SP tab, Glutammune Sachet, Mucinac 600mg, Nutrolin B Cap, Chemo and radiation therapy, PTCA (stenting).

Intervention (Diet Therapy) : The customized DIP diet plan was followed from 11-May-20 for 3 months and subsequently followed standard DIP Diet.

Outcome: After 6 months

Present Status : Overall condition improved, all symptoms and discomforts gone .

Discomforts: Nil

Ongoing Medicines: Brilinta 90mg , Rozucor ASP-20, Ativan 2mg

Life -saving W.I.S.E truth :

He was suffering for 8 years. Just compare the medicines he was taking before starting the DIP diet and the medicines now. The truth is; he doesn't need even those 3 medicines which he decided to continue.

2

Multiple myeloma & childhood asthma

Medical history of the patient at the time when he contacted us:

Ram Pratap Yadav, 69yrs from UP India contacted our office on 11 May 2020 through Virtual OPD/VOPD

Diagnosis: Multiple myeloma, bronchial asthma since childhood, asthmatic problem aggravated.

Discomforts: some reaction of medicine occurred so the whole body skin was infected and even skin from the sides of the nails were peeling off. feeling acute weakness couldn't move smoothly, acidity, constipation.

Medicines/ medical intervention: Inj Borviz 2gm, Weekly Chemo 16 Inj recommended 8 Inj Completed, Thalix: Ecosprin, Acyclovir 400mg, Flucon, Septran, Seroflo, Rotacap inhaler 4 times/Day .

Intervention (Diet Therapy) : The customized DIP diet plan was followed from 19-May-20 for 3 months subsequently followed by standard DIP Diet Plan till date.

Outcome: After 7 months

Present Status : Childhood asthma recovered a lot, inhaler usage reduced from 4 times/day to 2 times/day. Feeling very Good, weakness reduced, No more acidity, passing stools normally.

Discomforts: Nil

Medications: Inj Borviz 2gm weekly, Ecosprin, Acyclovir, Flucon, Septran, Rotacap inhaler 2 times a day

Life -saving W.I.S.E truth/ Analysis/ Analysis:

Greatly reduced symptoms/discomforts. Reduced medicines within 3 months of following DIP diet. Since it's a childhood disease, so full recovery is expected to happen by following the recommended diet for at least 1 year.

3

Peripheral Neuropathy, Prostate Enlargement, Diabetes & High BP

Medical history of the patient before he started the DIP diet:

Surjit Singh, 58 years, from Abu Dhabi, U.A.E

Diagnosis: Diabetes & Prostate Enlargement

Discomforts: High Blood Sugar readings, burning sensation in Feet, very less sensations in Feet, problems while passing urine.

Medicine/Intervention: Janumet 50/1000, Cafter Heels, Diamicron XR 60, Rozavel F 5, D- Rise 2000, Centrum Gold, Cardace 5 mg, PSA- 0.7ng/mL

Intervention (Diet Therapy): He started the DIP diet on his own after watching a viral video.

Outcome: After 3 Years now at the time of publishing this book

Present Status: Perfectly Fine, no more Feet Burning, Blood sugar readings are fine, now no issues while passing urine.

Discomforts: Nil

Medications: Nil

Life -saving W.I.S.E truth:

I was bewildered to see the blood report of one of the 105 patients, who joined our 3 days residential tour (27th to 29th April, 2018) as I could not find even a single parameter out of range. It was a recent medical report of perfectly healthy and dynamic gentleman, Mr. Surjit, who was on zero medication. I was curious to know why he came all the way from Abu Dhabi to join the residential tour in New Delhi.

It all started about 3 months back, when he happened to stumble upon one of my Youtube viral video "Blood Sugar Live Experiment", while he was casually scrolling through his WhatsApp messages. He immediately decided to follow the DIP diet (as explained in the video) and to his surprise he could reverse all the medical conditions, which he was suffering from, for more than 2 decades. He came to the residential tour just to thank me for getting back his health.

He went on to promote & propagate the DIP Diet by collaborating with the Indian Embassy in U.A.E and was later appointed as a brand ambassador of Indo-Vietnam Medical board during the annual convocation at Ho Chi Minh city, Vietnam, for his contribution in promoting DIP diet

4

Common Variable Immunodeficiency, Inflammatory Bowel Disease, Non-Cirrhotic Portal Fibrosis & Osteoporosis

Medical history of the patient at the time when he contacted us:

Ravi Raheja, 30yrs, from Maharashtra, India contacted us on 17 June 2020 through Virtual OPD/VOPD

Diagnosis: (CVID)Common Variable Immunodeficiency, IBD (tight rectal stricture) Severe Constipation, Non-Cirrhotic Portal Fibrosis, Osteoporosis.

Discomforts: Anxiety, fear and anxiety, breathlessness because of anxiety, heartbeat gets slow, severe constipation, severe pain in both legs.

Medicines/medical intervention: Immunoglobulins (IVIG) 25gMS, Saaz DS, Acotrust, Panlipase, Gemcal and seroflo250, Osteofos-35, Uprise-D3, homeopathic medicines

Intervention (Diet Therapy): The customized DIP diet plan was followed from 23-Jun-20 for 3 months and subsequently followed standard DIP Diet.

Outcome: After 6 months

Present Status: Constipation magically recovered, feeling light and good, being relieved, health issues have been cured by 80%.

Discomforts: Nil

Medications: Gemcal and Becasule plus.

Life -saving W.I.S.E truth:

It's a cocktail of a rare disease and dangerous medication. The patient recovered more than 80% after following the recommended diet for 6 months. Full recovery is expected by following the diet for about 4 months. The two medicines the patient decided to continue is not contributing in any way in improving his condition except giving him a psychological support.

5

Type 1 Diabetes with high insulin dosage

Medical history of the patient at the time when she contacted us:

Amena Wajahat, 20yrs, from Telangana, India contacted us on 20 June 2020 through Virtual OPD/VOPD

Diagnosis: Diabetes Type 1 with HbA1c-9.8%

Discomforts: Uneasiness in breathing, high blood sugar readings

Medicines/ medical intervention: 60U Insulin/day

Intervention (Diet Therapy) : The customized DIP diet plan was followed from 29-Jun-20 for 3 months and subsequently followed standard DIP Diet.

Outcome : After 6 months

Present Status: Sugar Readings < 200mg/dl HbA1c-8.5 %, left injecting insulin

Discomforts: NIL

Medications: NIL

Life -saving W.I.S.E truth:

The modern medical system will not dare to investigate the case study of Amena as she completed the unthinkable journey from being a Type 1 Diabetes patient with 60 unit of Insulin dependency to complete cure within just 6 months of following the DIP Diet, hence exposing the modern myth that once the beta cells are dead, cannot be regenerated.

6

Urgent Heart Bypass Surgery Advised & Angina

Medical history of the patient at the time when he contacted us :

Jasraj Suthar, 45yrs, from Telangana, India contacted us on 15 June 2020 through Virtual OPD/VOPD

Diagnosis: Heart problems, advised bypass surgery as soon as possible

Discomforts : Chest pain/angina

Medicines/medical intervention : Angioplasty 2 Stents implanted, Medicines include Polybion, Planep, Cardivas, Coversyl, Rosuvas, Duphalac, Sorbitrate, Rivotril, Korandil

Intervention (Diet Therapy) : The customized DIP diet plan was followed from 01-Jul-20 onwards till date

Outcome: After 6 months

Present Status: Bypass avoided, condition very much improved

Discomforts: Weight Loss - 73 Kg, low BP- 113/83

Medications: Coversyl

Life -saving W.I.S.E truth:

By avoiding bypass surgery not only he saved at least INR 5 lakh/- but also saved him of life- threatening side effects of bypass surgery. After losing weight and all other discomforts now it's time for him to get rid of the only medication which he is continuing.

7

Delusions, depression & high triglycerides

Medical history of the patient at the time when she contacted us:

Shameela Jameeli, 57yrs, from Cambridgeshire, United Kingdom contacted us on 27 March 2020 through Virtual OPD/VOPD.

Diagnosis: Delusions, depression & high triglycerides

Discomforts: Loss of appetite, irregular heartbeat.

Medicines: Aripiprazole 5mg, Atorvastatin 20mg

Intervention (Diet Therapy): The customized DIP diet plan was followed from 03-Apr-20 for 3 months and subsequently followed standard DIP Diet after 3 months.

Outcome: After 8 months

Present Status: Feeling energetic & happy, no depression, lost excess weight

Discomforts: Nil

Medications: Nil

Life -saving W.I.S.E truth:

Lost excess weight, lost all symptoms and discomforts. No surprise lost all medicines as well, as you must understand the medicine itself was the part of the problem.

8

Chronic Kidney Disease, Diabetes (Insulin Dependent), high BP & thyroid

Medical history of the patient at the time when he contacted us:

Mathura Singh Bisht, 69yrs, from New Delhi, India contacted us on 1 July 2020 through Virtual OPD/VOPD

Diagnosis: High Creatinine Kidneys Disease, Insulin Dependent Diabetic and BP TSH-2.77, Glucose fasting-130, glucose PP-150, triglyceride-202 mg/dl, HDL-33 mg/dl Serum Creatinine-2.23

Discomforts: Constipation

Medicines/ medical intervention: Humalog Insulin: 38 Units, Janumet 50/500mg) Abf Nebicard 5mg, Thyrox 25mg & 50mg, Prax A 10mg, Osucor10mg, Urimax .04mg, Fevujet 40mg, Angispan 2.6mg+ Dytor 5mg, Pantocid 40mg, Becosule, Homoeopathy Medicine + Nefrozon 500mg, Heart Surgery (2 Stents implanted), Thyroid Surgery (one gland removed)

Intervention (Diet Therapy) : The customized DIP diet plan was followed from 8 July 2020 and subsequently followed standard DIP Diet.

Outcome: After 5 months

Present Status: TSH-2.6, Glucose fasting-110, Glucose PP-130, Serum Creatinine- 1.4mg/dl

Discomforts: Nil

Medications: Prax, & Thyrox (alternate days)

Life -saving W.I.S.E truth:

High Dose of Insulin, high creatinine, 2 surgeries and about a dozen pills is what Mathura Singh was presented to us with, about 5 months back but now at the time of publishing this book, he has reversed all the medical conditions with negligible medication. This happened by adopting the recommended DIP Diet.

9

Rheumatoid Arthritis, Piles & Thyroid

Medical history of the patient at the time when she contacted us:

Savita Phogat, 45yrs, from Bahadurgarh Haryana, India contacted us on 25 June 2020 through Virtual OPD/VOPD

Diagnosis: Thyroid, Rheumatoid Arthritis, Piles, mind always in a state of confusion

Discomforts: pain in right knee, difficulty to get fresh in the morning, belly bloating, body weakness

Medicines/ medical intervention: Calcium, Medrol, Folitrax 20, Folvite 5, HCQs 300

Intervention (Diet Therapy): The customized DIP diet plan was followed from 05-Jul-20 for 3 months and subsequently followed standard DIP Diet.

Outcome: After 5 months

Present Status: excess-weight lost, belly fat reduced, active mind and body, grasping power increased, feeling good for almost everything.

Discomforts: Nil

Medication: Nil

Life -saving W.I.S.E truth/ Analysis:

With DIP diet, no disease is permanent as in this case in just 5 months got rid of 5 so called permanent illnesses.

10

Breast Cancer & High BP

Medical history of the patient at the time when she contacted us:

Kamlesh Kaur, 64yrs, from New Delhi, India contacted us on 21 Dec 2019 through Virtual OPD/VOPD

Diagnosis: Breast cancer stage 2, High BP

Discomforts: Nil

Medicines/ medical intervention: Nil

Intervention (Diet Therapy) : The customized DIP diet plan was followed from 01-Feb-20 and even after 10 months still following the customized DIP diet.

Outcome: After 10 months

Present Status : Lost unwanted 14 kg weight (from 82 kg to 68 kg), Lump in the breast- not increased, Energy level Good, BP level is normal

Discomforts: Nil

Medications: Nil

Life -saving W.I.S.E truth

Killing two flies with one slap - arresting the breast cancer, arresting high BP with just small modification in daily diet. Only thing which increased is energy level.

11

Thyroid, Hypertension, & High cholesterol

Medical history of the patient at the time when she contacted us:

Simta Manchanda, 64 yrs, from New Delhi, India contacted us on 2 July 2020 through Virtual OPD/VOPD

Diagnosis: Hypertension (level 165/90); High cholesterol; Thyroid

Discomforts: Waking up from deep sleep every night with severe headache, burning eyes and dried throat/mouth, coupled with high BP up to 165/90, Bloated stomach, Unable to sleep for more than 5-6 hours with disturbed sleep patterns every 1.5-2 hours.

Medicines/ medical intervention: Rosedays 10mg, Eslo 2.5mg, Trika 0.25mg, Concor 5mg & Natrilix SR Tablets, Thyroxine Sodium Tablets IP

Intervention (Diet Therapy): The customized DIP diet plan was followed from 3rd July onwards for 3 months and subsequently followed standard DIP Diet.

Outcome: After 5 months

Present Status: Headache is relieved, Dizziness is reduced, 1 kg weight lost.

Discomforts: Nil

Medications: Thyroxine 6.25 mg half tablet.

Life -saving W.I.S.E truth:

Waking up in the middle of the night with severe headache, hypertension and thyroid disease were some of the problems with which Simta contacted us. Now, after 5 months of following the DIP Diet, all the symptoms gone and also the dependency of medicines reduced drastically.

12

Advance stage Kidney Disease, Dialysis & High BP

Medical history of the patient at the time when he contacted us:

Jitendra Kumar, 44yrs, from Jharkhand, India contacted us on 3 August 2020 through Virtual OPD/VOPD

Diagnosis: CKD, Hypertension since 2014, Dialysis since 2018 (twice weekly).

Discomforts: Swelling in legs/faces, urine output is negligible, weakness/breathlessness while walking upstairs. High BP, low Hb (9.3), insomnia, vomiting tendency during morning mouth cleaning (tooth brushing), High PTH (900)

Medicines/ medical intervention: Nicaradia 20, Staha 5, Bio D3, Nexiron LP, Sevlaren 400, Inj. Zyrop 10000, Inj. Ferinject 100

Intervention (Diet Therapy): The customized DIP diet plan was followed from 13-Aug-20 till date

Outcome: After 4 months

Present Status: Now Dialysis reduced to just once in 5 days.

Discomforts: Nil

Medications: Staha 5

Life -saving W.I.S.E truth

Advance stage of kidney disease, dialysis twice a week and list of medicines & injections was the status of Jitendra 4 months back. Now after following the DIP diet for 4 months he got rid of all the injections and most of the medicines and also dialysis requirement reduced to half. Hope to be free of dialysis in the next 4 months.

13

Lung Cancer & high BP

Medical history of the patient at the time when she contacted us:

Nirmala Gupta, 54yrs, from Rewari, Haryana, India contacted us on 15 August 2020 through Virtual OPD/VOPD

Diagnosis: Lung Cancer, high BP

Discomforts: Fluid retention in the lungs, on oxygen cylinder, oxygen level between 90-95

Medicines/ medical intervention: Tab. Gefitinib, Inj Clexane, Cap Pantocid, Tab Zerodol

Intervention (Diet Therapy): The customized DIP diet plan was followed from 14-Aug-20 for 3 months and subsequently following standard DIP Diet.

Outcome: After 4 months

Present Status: Feeling Better in every sense

Discomforts: Nil

Medications: Clexane 60mg/ 0.6 Ml Nurokind Lc, Gefitinib 250 Mg

Life -saving W.I.S.E truth/ Analysis:

In just 4 months major symptom relieved and can escape from life threatening and deadly medicines which the patient is continuing because of her long-held belief that the medicine has a role in cure.

14

Angina & acid reflux

Medical history of the patient at the time when he contacted us:

Vivekanand Labhane, 55yrs, from Maharashtra, India contacted us on 20 August 2020 through Virtual OPD

Diagnosis: Chest pain, Headache, Discomfort (specifically in throat), Acidity/acid reflux & Sleeplessness

Discomforts: continuous chest pain (in the afternoon it increases), headache, discomfort in throat, acid reflux & sleeplessness.

Medicines/ medical intervention: Paxidep cr 12.5 mg, ELM cr 1.5 mg and Homeopathic medicines

Intervention (Diet Therapy): The customized DIP diet plan was followed from 29-Aug-20 for 3 months and subsequently followed standard DIP Diet.

Outcome: After 4 months

Present Status: 80% relief in acid reflux, stomach pain, no headache

Discomforts: Nil

Medications: ELM 0.5 mg at night (reduced dose).

Life -saving W.I.S.E truth

Chest Pain normally interpreted as angina, a precursor to heart attack, is what with which Vivekanand contacted us while having several other health issues as well . We contacted him just before the printing of the book to know that he is free of all symptoms and is on negligible medicines while following the DIP diet for 4 months now

15

Diabetes Type 2 (Insulin dependent) & anxiety

Medical history of the patient at the time when he contacted us:

Ashutosh, 20 yrs, from Chandigarh, India contacted us on 15 September 2020 through Virtual OPD/VOPD

Diagnosis: Diabetes type 2 (insulin dependent)

Discomforts: Anxiety after eating dinner

Medicines/ medical intervention: 5 Unit of Insulin and taking homeopathic Medicines- Jambolanum Q, Chirata Q, Gymnema Q, Cephalandra Q

Intervention (Diet Therapy): The customized DIP diet plan was followed from 20-Sep-20 onwards till date.

Outcome: After 3 months

Present Status: All symptoms vanished and readings are in normal range very happy and energy levels are high.

Discomforts: Nil

Medications: Nil

Life -saving W.I.S.E truth:

A cocktail of homeopathic medicine and insulin with which Ashutosh was trying to control his blood sugar before contacting us. Now after 3 months of following the DIP diet, he is free of all medicine/insulin and also all symptoms vanished.

16

Chronic Kidney Disease with low urine output

Medical history of the patient at the time when he contacted us:

Dharam Singh, 42 yrs, from M.P, India contacted us on 1 June 2020 through Virtual OPD/VOPD

Diagnosis: Chronic kidney Disease with Creatinine:1.77 & GFR-43ml/min/1.73m2

Discomforts: Body Pain, Pain in Knees, feeling fatigued, Burning sensation in eyes, Burning sensation in urine, problems while passing urine, urine output decreased.

Medicines/ medical intervention: Nil

Intervention (Diet Therapy): The customized DIP diet plan was followed from 23-Jun-20 for 3 months and subsequently followed standard DIP Diet.

Outcome: After 6 months.

Present Status: Creatinine is lowered to 1.6, urea also reduced, uric acid 6.1, platelets improved

Discomforts: Fatigued

Medications: Nil

Life -saving W.I.S.E truth:

After following the DIP diet for 6 months Dharam Singh could get rid of most of the symptoms and was also able to reduce the creatinine to a near normal range

17

Dermatomyositis

Medical history of the patient at the time when she contacted us:

Rinku Goyal, 48yrs, from West Bengal, India contacted us on 14 May 2020 through Virtual OPD/VOPD

Diagnosis: Dermatomyositis

Discomforts: Nil

Medicines/ medical intervention: Wysolone 7.5, Folitrax 15mg, Folvite 5mg, Cardace 5mg, Shelcal 500mg, Calcirol Sachet 60K, Inj Mabtas RA 500mg

Intervention (Diet Therapy): The customized DIP diet plan was followed from 18-May-20 for 3 months & subsequently followed standard DIP Diet.

Outcome: After 7 months

Present Status: feeling very good, stopped all the medicines

Discomforts: Nil

Medications: nil

Life -saving W.I.S.E truth:

Struggling to cure dermatomyositis with the combination of drugs and injection, Rinku, decided to adopt the DIP diet. Now after7 months, she is free of all medicines and all the symptoms as well.

18

Heart Disease & Diabetes

Medical history of the patient at the time when he contacted us:

Debashish Bhattacharya, 58yrs, from Tripura, India contacted us on 8 September 2020 through Virtual OPD/VOPD

Diagnosis: Heart Disease, Diabetes

Discomforts: acidity, gas, constipation, indigestion, nausea, body pain, skin problems, sleeplessness, uneasy

Medicines/ medical intervention: Cardivas 3.125, Renerve plus, Ecosprin, Gemer1 and Glycomet500

Intervention (Diet Therapy): The customized DIP diet plan was followed from 12-Sep-20 for 3 months and subsequently followed standard DIP Diet.

Outcome: After 3 months

Present Status: 100% healthy

Discomforts: Nil

Medications: Nil

Life -saving W.I.S.E truth:

Debashish Bhattacharya contacted us with a long list of discomforts and a history of heart disease and diabetes. However, within 4 months of following the prescribed DIP Diet, all his symptoms vanished and also, he stopped consuming all medicines.

19

Brain Tumor

Medical history of the patient at the time when she contacted us:

Meenakshi Sharma, 24yrs, from New Delhi, India contacted us on 18 September 2020 through Virtual OPD/VOPD

Diagnosis: Brain Tumor

Discomforts: Headache, no periods for the last 1.5 years, not able to see properly from right eye.

Medicines/ medical intervention: Nil

Intervention (Diet Therapy): The customized DIP diet plan was followed from 26-Sep-20 for 3 months and subsequently following standard DIP Diet.

Outcome: After 4 months

Present Status: Feeling better than earlier, vision improved

Discomforts: Periods yet not started

Medications: Nil

Life -saving W.I.S.E truth

It's an eye-opening testimonial with the eye sight improvement which may be an unimaginable fact by the present mainstream medicine. It may take another 4 months on DIP diet to get back her regular menstrual cycle.

20

25% Heart working

Medical history of the patient at the time when he contacted us:

Mahesh Kumar Taneja, 65yrs, from Haryana, India contacted us on 25 August 2020 through Virtual OPD/VOPD

Diagnosis: Heart is damaged and working 25%

Discomforts: Breathlessness, High BP, excessive urination, general weakness, loss of weight and muscles, stomach upset unable to climb stairs.

Medicines/ medical intervention: Tab. Clavix Gold, Cap Pan D, Tab Embeta XR, Tab Alprax 0.25, Tab Vymada 50, Tab Flavedon MR,Tab Dytor 10, Eptus 25mg

Intervention (Diet Therapy): The customized DIP diet plan was followed from 01-Sep-20 for 3 months and subsequently followed standard DIP Diet.

Outcome: After 3 months

Present Status: Now heart is 45-50 % working. Can climb stairs without any discomfort.

Discomforts: Nil

Medications: Nil

Life -saving W.I.S.E truth:

100% improvement in heart condition with zero percent medicine and zero discomfort, that too within 3 months of following the DIP diet.

21

Rheumatoid Arthritis, Thyroid & heart diseases

Medical history of the patient at the time when she contacted us:

Asha Prasad, 66 yrs, from Jharkhand, India contacted us on 24 July 2020 through Virtual OPD/VOPD

Diagnosis: Rheumatoid Arthritis, Thyroid, heart attack

Discomforts: Chest pain, Back pain, breathing problems, extreme weakness, not feeling hunger, constipation, joint pain due to Rheumatoid Arthritis, unshaped bone of hand and feet fingers.

Medicines/ medical intervention: Folic acid, Sazo, Hydroxy Chloroquine, Ibandronic acid, Methotrexate 15mg, Thyronorm, Orthosol tablets, Deplatt a 75mg, Atorva 40mg, Ramfirst, Inj MS5. Inj fondum 2.5mg, Tramadol, Injection Cefokem XP, Inj. Lasix 20, Tab Ivanode, Inj Norad, Ativan,Inj Neurokind gold, Syp. Emty 15mg, Syp. Alkasol Syp, Phensedy l-LR 10ml

Intervention (Diet Therapy): The customized DIP diet plan was followed from 30-Jul-20 for 3 months and subsequently followed standard DIP Diet.

Outcome: After 5 months

Present Status: All discomfort related to cardiac vanished. There is arthritis pain at times but handling it without any allopathic medicine or pain killer

Discomforts: Nil

Medications: Nil

Life -saving W.I.S.E truth:

Journey from 15 medicines to zero medicines within 5 months of following the DIP diet may look like a miracle but is a common phenomenon among our patients.

22

Diabetes (Insulin Dependent)

Medical history of the patient at the time when she contacted us :

Rajini M Kumar, 49 yrs, from Bangalore, India contacted us on 1st August 2020 through Virtual OPD/VOPD

Diagnosis: Diabetes with sugar readings between 234mg/dl to 421mg/dl

Discomforts: High readings, Frozen shoulder

Medicines/medical intervention: Insulin 38 Units & Homoeopathic medicines

Intervention (Diet Therapy): The customized DIP diet plan was followed from 06-Aug-20 for 3 months and subsequently followed standard DIP Diet.

Outcome: After 4 months

Present Status: The blood glucose levels have improved to a very great extent 144 mg/dl to 156 mg/dl

Discomforts: Nil

Medications: Nil

Life -saving W.I.S.E truth:

Initially on Homeopathic medicine, then Insulin and still uncontrollably high blood sugar is what defines Rajini till she decided to adopt DIP Diet. Now after 5 months of following the recommended DIP Diet, she is free of Insulin / medicine and is able to maintain blood sugar in a healthy range.

23

Gastritis & Thyroid

Medical history of the patient at the time when she contacted us:

K. Bhargavi, 29yrs, from Chennai, India contacted us on 7 August 2020 through Virtual OPD/VOPD

Diagnosis: Thyroid, Gastric Problem (Burping, Gas Pain, Back Pain Leg Pain), Hair fall and general weakness of body

Discomforts: Gastric problems like frequent burping, gas, pain in legs hands, knees, and body pain like hip pain, back pain, and general weakness in the body and numbness of hands and legs while napping even for a short time, severe hair fall

Medicines/medical intervention: Thyronorm - 25mg, Kanchanara Guggulu and Chitra Grantikadi Kashayam.

Intervention (Diet Therapy): The customized DIP diet plan was followed from 18-Aug-20 for 3 months and subsequently followed standard DIP Diet.

Outcome: After 4 months

Present Status: Thyroid value has reduced, gastric problem is reduced very much, and my body pain has also reduced, feeling very active and energetic throughout the day.

Discomforts: Nil

Medications: Nil

Life -saving W.I.S.E truth:

Two mutually exclusive medical conditions and a lot of discomforts, is what with which K. Bhargavi contacted us, now after more than 4 months of following the prescribed DIP Diet, she is free of drugs and disease fully.

24

Diabetes & Thyroid

Medical history of the patient at the time when she contacted us:

Surekha Habib, 49 yrs, from Karnataka,India contacted us on 2 September 2020 through Virtual OPD/VOPD

Diagnosis: Diabetes, Blood Pressure (Normal but advised to take Tablet), right leg great toe amputation, Thyroid, acidity problem, right eye issue, Irregular mensuration, frequent Motion, no sound sleep

Discomforts: Acidity problem, Heartburn, Frequent Motions, Leg pain till thigh after operation, Knee pain.

Medicines/ medical intervention: Glimisave MF 2/500, Gemer, Gluvida M 500, Olkem 20 AM, Ultracet Nurokind 100mg, Pan -D, Duonem 200mg, Kanchana Guggal.

Intervention (Diet Therapy): The customized DIP diet plan was followed from 11-Sep-20 for 3 months and subsequently followed standard DIP Diet.

Outcome: After 3 months

Present Status: Weight loss & feeling better health

Discomforts: Nil

Medications: Gemer 3 but not every day.

Life -saving W.I.S.E truth:

Toe amputation, more than ½ dozen medical conditions and high doses of a handful of pills is what defines Surekha till she started the DIP Diet. Now after 3 months she is free of all major medical issues and medication dependency reached to near negligible.

25

Retroperitoneal neoplasm

Medical history of the patient at the time when he contacted us:

Dileep Singh, 35yrs, from U.P, India contacted us on 25 September 2020 through Virtual OPD/VOPD

Diagnosis: Retroperitoneal neoplasm

Discomforts: Stomach pain, swelling and feeling of something stuck in the stomach.

Medicines/ medical intervention: Omega 3 capsule per day

Intervention (Diet Therapy): The customized DIP diet plan was followed from 25-Sep-20 for 3 months and subsequently followed standard DIP Diet.

Outcome: After 3 months

Present Status: Size of tumor/lesion is same, pains relieved to a great extent

Discomforts: Pains rarely

Medications: Nil

Life -saving W.I.S.E truth:

A rare disease in control within 3 months of following DIP diet, expected to remain symptom free lifelong if avoid any further invasive diagnosis with strict adherence to the DIP diet.

26

Prostate enlargement, dry eyes & High BP

Medical history of the patient at the time when he contacted us:

Satyajit Thakur, 66yrs, from UP, India contacted us on 28 June 2020 through Virtual OPD/VOPD

Diagnosis: High BP, slight difficulty in breathing while fast walk, prostate enlargement, right ear deaf since childhood, dry eye, left hand weak and muscle loss, teeth decay.

Discomforts: Bone pain in legs, jerking and trembling, no free flow of urine, takes longer time in the morning for complete evacuation with burning pain. Right eye - sometimes more tear flow. During morning and evening tears ooze from right eye.

Medicines/ medical intervention: Sartel beta 25mg, ecosprin, Urimax 0.4gm/tamsulosin0.4mg Vit.D3 calciquickD3, Systane ultra-eye drop, Glycol 0.3% drop/glyvisc lubricant eye drop

Intervention (Diet Therapy): The customized DIP diet plan was followed from 02-Jul-20 for 3 months and subsequently followed standard DIP Diet.

Outcome: After 5 months

Present Status: Feeling light and energetic, sound sleep body pain reduced, fat reduced.

Discomforts: Weight loss

Medications: Nil

Life -saving W.I.S.E truth

Major relief from multiple discomforts and total freedom from all the medicines in just 5 months of following the DIP diet. A long-term DIP diet may bring back complete life to the childhood right ear deafness.

27

Uncontrolled Diabetes & High BP

Medical history of the patient at the time when he contacted us:

Umesh chandra Goswami, 65yrs, from Jharkhand,India contacted us on 15 September 2020 through Virtual OPD/VOPD

Diagnosis: Diabetes and High Blood Pressure from 13 years, fever and weakness

Discomforts: Fever, too much weakness and sugar level 280 and BP-150/85

Medicines/ medical intervention: Prichek M2 Forte, Prichek M1, Concor 2.5, Losar 50 & Amlosafe 5, A to Z Tablet, Ruby-DSR 1 Tablet

Intervention (Diet Therapy): 3 step Flu Diet was followed for 3 days for fever followed by the customized DIP diet plan from 22-Sep-20.

Outcome: After 3 months

Present Status: Sugar level and blood pressure has been normal and feeling more energetic than earlier

Discomforts: Nil

Medications: Nil

Life -saving W.I.S.E truth:

Fever along with co-morbid condition of a 65 years old Patient, can be easily seen as a life-threatening situation especially in this Coronakaal, however for Umesh Chandra Goswami, it had been a smooth journey to recovery after he started the recommended 3 step flu Diet followed by the DIP Diet, now after 3 months, he is free of all medicines and all complications as well.

28

Pulmonary Malfunction, Low SpO2 & abnormally high Hemoglobin

Medical history of the patient at the time when he contacted us:

Raghvendra singh, 7 yrs, from Bangalore, India contacted us on 15 July 2020 through Virtual OPD/VOPD

Diagnosis: Pulmonary Malfunction in Left Lung SpO_2: 80-81%, High Hemoglobin -22

Discomforts: Headache and nausea in the morning, dizziness

Medicines/ medical intervention: Pentoxifylill, Nodosis

Intervention (Diet Therapy): The customized DIP diet plan was followed from 22-Jul-20 for 3 months and subsequently followed standard DIP Diet.

Outcome: After 5 months

Present Status: SpO_2 - 85-86%, Hemoglobin reduced to 20

Discomforts: Nil

Medications: Nil

Life -saving W.I.S.E truth:

Rarest of the rare disease with high hemoglobin and low SPO_2, is in the path of fast paced recovery within a few months of following the DIP Diet.

29

Rheumatoid arthritis

Medical history of the patient at the time when she contacted us:

Simran Handa 44yrs, from Karnal, Haryana contacted us on 22 July 2020 through Virtual OPD/VOPD/VOPD

Diagnosis: Rheumatoid arthritis

Discomforts: Extreme rheumatic joint and muscle pain, neck pain, pinched vein. Frequent bowel movements in a day.

Medicines/medical intervention: Methotrexate 20mg, Leflunomide 10, Folvite 5 mg, Calcirol 60000 IU/gm, injection Depo Medrol 80mg

Intervention (Diet Therapy): The customized DIP diet plan was followed from 28-Jul-20 for 3 months and subsequently followed standard DIP Diet.

Outcome: After 5 months

Present Status: 70 - 80% relief in pain, weight loss (was 63kg and now, 58 kg), higher energy levels.

Discomforts: Nil

Medications: Nil

Life -saving W.I.S.E truth

Zero medicine and 70-80% relief within just 5 months of following the DIP Diet. Her Case is a cocktail of illness & discomforts which normally continues lifelong if the patient plans to stick to allopathic medicine .

30

Rectal Cancer & Diabetes

Medical history of the patient at the time when he contacted us:

Bind Prabhuram, 49yrs, from Gujrat, India contacted us on 18 June 2020 through Virtual OPD/VOPD

Diagnosis: Malignant melanoma cancer in rectum, Sugar

Discomforts: One node outside the rectum causing pain.

Medicines/ medical intervention: Granisetron, Dacarbazine, Dexamethasone, Nivolumab

Intervention (Diet Therapy): The customized DIP diet plan was followed from 23-Jun-20 for 3 months and subsequently followed standard DIP Diet.

Outcome: After 6 months

Present Status: outer cancerous node size decreased by 35%, no pain

Discomforts: Nil

Medications: Nivolumab

Life -saving W.I.S.E truth

With almost Zero medication and zero discomforts, it's a great recovery within just 6 months of following the DIP Diet.

31

Peripheral Neuropathy & Diabetes

Medical history of the patient at the time when he contacted us:

Harpal Singh, 38yrs, from Ontario, Canada contacted us on 12 September 2020 through Virtual OPD/VOPD

Diagnosis: Diabetes with average sugar readings 16mmol (288mg/dl)

Discomforts: Head is too heavy feels like a belt / rock in the middle, dizziness while sittings over the toilet seat, chest pain in upper left side, numbness in right thumb feet for the last 1 year, getting tired quickly.

Medicines/ medical intervention: Heart bypass surgery in Feb-2019. Medications left a few days before taking Virtual OPD/ VOPD as they started DIP diet from online videos.

Intervention (Diet Therapy): The customized DIP diet plan was followed from 23-Sep-20 till date Still following 98% diet plan without any cheating day.

Outcome: After 3 months

Present Status: Average sugar levels dropped to 9.4 mmol. right foot thumb numbness gone, energy level is very good, not feeling sleepy anymore, not feeling regular dizziness like before while sitting down or bending legs on the toilet seat.

Discomforts: Nil

Medications: Nil

Life -saving W.I.S.E truth

After the bypass surgery with uncontrolled blood sugar and a long list of discomfort was the time when Harpal came to know about the DIP diet through a Youtube video, in the month of August 2020. He decided to stop all the medicines and strictly follow the DIP diet. Now at the time of the book going into the press, he is free from all symptoms and discomforts and also never wants back to medicines.

32

Throat Cancer

Medical history of the patient at the time when she contacted us:

Rajbala, 47 yrs, from Rajasthan, India contacted us on 7 August 2020 through Virtual OPD/VOPD

Diagnosis: Throat Cancer

Discomforts: Throat pain

Medicines/ medical intervention: Omnicef, Am Gargle, Esocare LSR, Zerodol–P

Intervention (Diet Therapy): The customized DIP diet plan was followed from 13-Aug-20 for 3 months and subsequently followed standard DIP Diet.

Outcome: After 4 months

Present Status: No discomforts, no throat pain.

Discomforts: Nil

Medications: Nil

Life -saving W.I.S.E truth

Throat Cancer, known to be a Painful disease, often ends with the death of a patient, but luckily for Rajbala, she decided to tread an unconventional path of DIP Diet as a result within 4 months, she is free of medicines and suffering.

33

Chronic Kidney Disease, Diabetes (high insulin dependency

Medical history of the patient at the time when she contacted us:

Ishrat khan, 66yrs, from Maharashtra, India contacted us on 1 Dec 2019 through Virtual OPD/VOPD

Diagnosis: CKD, Diabetes, High Creatinine 7.5

Discomforts: Uncontrolled diabetes, Creatinine 7.5, blood Urea 224, problem in passing stool, weakness while working.

Medicines/ medical intervention: Insulin- 120 Units, Tab Roseday A 10/75, Tab Febuget 40, Tab. Laretol, Tab.Efonta,Tab Aldactone, Tab Thyronorm, Cap.Nephrocap, Tab Sonaxa Nt, Tab Amaryl, Tab Zytanix, Tab Meltor, Tab Semi Ultracet, Tab Rebonah Dsr, Tab Fevpar 400mg, Tab Prazopress Xl Tab Concor 2.5, Tab Effonta 40mg

Intervention (Diet Therapy): The customized DIP diet plan was followed from 05-Dec-19 for 3 months and subsequently followed standard DIP Diet.

Outcome: After 1 year

Present Status: Creatinine level 5.5, Blood Urea -113, Good Sugar Level, Good Blood Pressure.

Discomforts: Nil

Medications: BP Medicine 10 mg occasionally out of fear

Life -saving W.I.S.E truth:

With very high creatinine, about 2 dozen pills and 120 units of 2 types of insulin Ishrat khan contacted us a year back. Now after one year of following the DIP Diet, she is free of all the symptoms and got rid of Insulin and just as a matter if habit continuing with the unnecessary B.P medicine.

34

Ulcerative colitis, & Migraine

Medical history of the patient at the time when she contacted us:

Bharati Bhushan Patel, 42yrs, from Pune, India contacted us on 1 October 2020 through Virtual OPD/VOPD

Diagnosis: Ulcerative colitis, Migraine

Discomforts: Bleeding and pain in colon, severe headache

Medicines/ medical intervention: Asacus 2mg, Azoran 50, Shelcal 500, Folvit, Wysolin,

Intervention (Diet Therapy): The customized DIP diet plan was followed from 09-Oct-20 for 2 months and still being continued.

Outcome: After 2 months

Present Status: Feeling Good

Discomforts: Nil

Medications: Nil

Life -saving W.I.S.E truth

Ulcerative colitis and migraine are the kind of diseases that last lifetime for most of the patients but for Bharti Bhushan, just 2 months of DIP Diet resulted in freedom from the disease, drugs and doctors as well.

35

Epilepsy

Medical history of the patient at the time when he contacted us:

Rishabh (name changed), 7yrs, from Tamil Nadu, India contacted us on 21 August 2020 through Virtual OPD/VOPD

Diagnosis: Epilepsy

Discomforts: Gets spikes daily which lasts for 2 seconds (sometimes he gets less than 5 times a day, sometimes it will be 20 times or even more) – there will be eye roll, EEG reports show he gets such spikes in sleep too, Mild shaky hands. Sometimes loss of appetite and mild nausea (week to 10 days, once in 45 days), Poor stamina, by afternoon his eyes get dark circles and he becomes dull, Slow grasping or learning skills, before seizures he was very quick in learning, Unable to communicate fluently, he faces difficulty in choosing words to express himself, his weight and height has not increased.

Medicines/ medical intervention: Valparin 200 syrup 5ml, Frisium 5mg, Topamax 25mg

Intervention (Diet Therapy): The customized DIP diet plan was followed from 27-Aug-20 for 3 months and subsequently followed standard DIP Diet.

Outcome: After 4 months

Present Status: Within a week of following the DIP diet & stopping the medicines found him active, jumping and running around in the house, studies, focus, attention span improved, better at communication, appetite increased

Discomforts: eye rolling still persists.

Medications: Stopped all medicines

Life -saving W.I.S.E truth

Most of the epilepsy patients are given unproven and unscientific treatment protocol, which are often more damaging than the disease itself. But for this 7-year-old child just 4 months of DIP Diet led to the total transformation in his physical and mental well-being and also got rid of all the medicines on the day of starting the diet.

36

Chronic kidney Disease

Medical history of the patient at the time when he contacted us:

Faizur Rahman, 57yrs, from Guwahati, India contacted us on 1 March 2020 through Virtual OPD/VOPD

Diagnosis: Chronic kidney Disease

Discomforts: Shortness of breath while climbing stairs, foam in urine, leg swelling, weight loss and weakness Medicines/medical intervention: Avastin injection, Sobisis Forte, Geroz LP, Nicardia Retard 20, Met XL50, Prazopress XL 2.5 mg, Eprex 4000 IU, Renokit, Acutrol C-400, Genevac-B Vaccine, Prevnar 13 Inj

Intervention (Diet Therapy): The customized DIP diet plan was followed from 08-Mar-20 for 3 months and subsequently followed standard DIP Diet.

Outcome: After 9 months

Present Status: Blood Pressure medicines have been reduced from 20mg to 10 mg. Creatinine was 5.2 on the 20th Aug 2020 report. It was reduced to 4.8 on the 31st Oct 2020 report. Hemoglobin was 7.3 on the 20th Aug 2020 report. It has increased to 8.0 on 31st Oct 2020 report.

Discomforts: Nil

Medications: 2 BP medications Prazopress &Nicardia

Life -saving W.I.S.E truth

Beside clinical achievement of reducing the creatinine level, increasing the hemoglobin level & better control on blood pressure, he could get rid of all the symptoms within 9 months of following the DIP diet.

37

Diabetes Type 1

Medical history of the patient at the time when he/she contacted us:

Shaurya Singh, 12yrs, from UP, India contacted us on 12 June 2020 through Virtual OPD/VOPD

Diagnosis: Diabetes type 1

Discomforts: Nil

Medicines/ medical intervention: Insulin Humalog and Lantus-22U

Intervention (Diet Therapy): The customized DIP diet plan was followed from 18-Jun-20 for 3 months and subsequently followed standard DIP Diet.

Outcome: After 6 months

Present Status: Sugar readings normalized

Discomforts: Nil

Medications: Nil

Life -saving W.I.S.E truth

Curing Diabetes type 1 may be an impossible fear for modern medicine, but is a common outcome for most of our type 1 children. Shaurya is one such case. Now it is over 6 months being on the DIP Diet, he is free of insulin and free of all complications, whatsoever.

38

Irritable bowel syndrome

Medical history of the patient at the time when she contacted us:

Sujana Jampani, 40yrs, from Secunderabad, India contacted us on through Virtual OPD/VOPD

Diagnosis: Irritable bowel syndrome

Discomforts: Vomiting sensation, frequent motion, gas, stomach bloating

Medicines/ medical intervention: Rifagut 200mg BD, Vibact DS BD, Colospa BD, Folvite BD, Methylcobalamin OD

Intervention (Diet Therapy): The customized DIP diet plan was followed from 15-Jan-20 for 3 months and subsequently followed standard DIP Diet.

Outcome: After 11 months

Present Status: Completely Healthy

Discomforts: No discomfort

Medications: Nil

Life -saving W.I.S.E truth

IBS is often accepted as a lifelong companion for most of the patients, but for Sujana, it's a full stop for IBS and all medications with the adoption of the DIP Diet

39

Rheumatic heart disease, severe aortic regurgitation, mild mitral regurgitation

Medical history of the patient at the time when he contacted us:

Deepak Mahato, 41yrs, from West Bengal, India contacted us on 1 January 2020 through Virtual OPD/VOPD

Diagnosis: Rheumatic heart disease, moderately severe aortic regurgitation, mild mitral regurgitation, eye cataract

Discomforts: Fatigue, Problem in climbing stairs.

Medicines/ medical intervention: Losanorm-H 50mg, Nebicard 2.5mg, Injection Penidure 12 Lakh Im

Intervention (Diet Therapy): The customized DIP diet plan was followed from 5th January 20 for 3 months and subsequently followed standard DIP Diet.

Outcome: After 11 months

Present Status: Feeling good & healthy

Discomforts: Cataract reduced but still persists

Medications: Nil

Life -saving W.I.S.E truth

A life-threatening heart disease and a deadly injection Penidure, is a suicidal combination. Deepak could escape both with DIP Diet. As a side benefit, he got improved vision and is on his way, to get rid of cataract as well. For speedy recovery from cataract, we suggest a specialized 15-minute exercise for 3-4 months which sometimes patients forget to continue, resulting in slower speed of recovery.

40

Kidney Disease & extremely high creatinine

Medical history of the patient at the time when she contacted us:

Pradnya Dusare, 41yrs from Madhya Pradesh, India contacted us on 10th Jun,2020 through Virtual OPD/VOPD

Diagnosis: Kidney problem, Creatinine level rise to 15, blood urea goes to 126.

Discomforts: Patient unable to do routine work, body got swollen, vomiting of food taken, no proper sleep at night

Medicines/ medical intervention: Concor 2.5, K K Wati, Chandraprabha vati, Punarnavasav, LIV-a GAIN

Intervention (Diet Therapy): The customized DIP diet plan was followed for 3 months and subsequently followed standard DIP Diet.

Outcome: After 6 months

Present Status: Good improvement, creatinine reduced to 5 from 15.

Discomforts: Sometimes BP rises, Back Pain

Medications: Cetanil M50, Haemoglobin Darbepoetin alfa injection 40 mcg once in a month.

Life -saving W.I.S.E truth

Besides a Great leap from creatinine 15 to 5, another achievement of Pradnya is getting rid of all the major discomforts which included inability to do routine work etc. All this could be achieved by sincerely following the customized DIP Diet

41

Primary pulmonary hypertension

Medical history of the patient at the time when he contacted us:

Aayush Srivastava, 30yrs, from U.P, India contacted us on 15 June 2020 through Virtual OPD/VOPD

Diagnosis: Primary pulmonary hypertension (PPH) or Primary arterial hypertension (PAH)

Discomforts: SPO_2 level 90, Physical activity limited in the winter season, needs oxygen cylinder for coughing and cold, running, cycle riding, climbing and other physical activities are not possible except walking, blood thick, frequent urination. Any physical activity causes low blood pressure and fainting, joint pain and swelling, chest pain, weakness

Medicines/ medical intervention: Ambrican 5 mg, Pulmopres 20 mg, Acitrom 4 mg, tide 20

Intervention (Diet Therapy): The customized DIP diet plan was followed from 23-Jun-20 for 3 months and subsequently followed standard DIP Diet.

Outcome: After 6 months

Present Status: Good improvement, Spo2 level never less than 93 % now

Discomforts: Nil

Medications: Nil

Life -saving W.I.S.E truth

Living with an oxygen cylinder and low SpO2 level can be very scary and worrisome. Aayush could not only get rid of all medications and oxygen cylinder after starting the DIP Diet, but could also maintain a healthy SpO2 level.

42

Heart Disease & Angina

Medical history of the patient at the time when he contacted us:

Sachin Patel, 41 yrs, from New Jersey, USA contacted us on 23 July 2020 through Virtual OPD/VOPD

Diagnosis: Heart Disease & Angina

Discomforts: Pain and tingling sensation in right arm, chest pressure, pain at the corner of left chest

Medicines/ medical intervention: Brilinta 90mg, Baby Aspirin, Metoprolol 12.5mg

Intervention (Diet Therapy): The customized DIP diet plan was followed from 31-Jul-20 for 3 months and subsequently followed standard DIP Diet.

Outcome: After 5 months

Present Status : Breathing is better and no pain in the chest area.

Discomforts: Nil

Medications: Nil

Life -saving W.I.S.E truth

Angina, often seen as a hint of the future heart attack, is what Sachin was scared of, till he contacted us through our website (www.biswaroop.com). Now it had been more than 5 months, since he started DIP Diet, He is free of all the symptoms including angina and also free of all medicines as well.

43

Advance Parkinson Disorder, Diabetes & High BP

Medical history of the patient at the time when he contacted us:

Umakant Dureja, 55yrs, from Gurugram, Haryana contacted us on 20 August 2020 through Virtual OPD/VOPD

Diagnosis: Advance Parkinson Disorder, Diabetes, High BP

Discomforts: Cannot blink eyes frequently, facial expressions do not change while talking, face appears like a mask, cough but unable to take out cough himself, low volume voice, speech is not clear, freezing and stiffness in entire body (eyes, mouth, tongue, upper and lower limbs (toes), tremors in the left hand and both the legs, slowness in entire body, forward bend posture, major constipation, catheter implanted since June 2019 and develops UTI every month, poor body balance, falls due to loss of balance, difficulty in swallowing, excessive salivation which keeps drooling from the half open mouth sometimes, currently unable to walk and perform daily activities himself. dependent on family members completely, can eat food only after taking levodopa medicine, short breath, running nose, watery eyes when having food, umbilical hernia

Medicines/medical intervention: Syndopa Plus, Janumet, Niftran, Livogen, Vigor, UTI Antibiotics, Arsenic Album

Intervention (Diet Therapy): The customized DIP diet plan was followed from 24-Aug-20 for 3 months and subsequently followed standard DIP Diet.

Outcome: After 4 months

Present Status: Diabetes (under 250) and BP under control. (120 +-5/80+-5), able to Blink eyes properly. Facial expressions are improving. The patient is now able to give expressions like laugh, low volume voice but speech is getting improved. 10% improvement seen in speech clarity, no Stiffness in entire body, patient is able to move his neck, hands on his own 10 % improvement, hardly any tremors seen, body balance improved by 15%, no constipation, no UTI, able to swallow food, no running nose.

Discomforts: Nil

Medications: Syndopa Plus.

Life -saving W.I.S.E truth

No constipation, no UTI, no running nose, no discomfort in swallowing, no stiffness in body, no diabetes, no hypertension, negligible medicine and a great recovery from advance stage of Parkinson and all of it in just 5 months with just one intervention 'The DIP diet'.

44

Cancerous Tumor & Osteoporosis

Medical History of the patient:

Simi Handa, Age: 55 years from New Delhi

Diagnosis: Cancer, Osteoporosis (-6)

Discomforts: Bedridden for one whole year due to Osteoporosis followed by walking with the help of crutches and walker

Medicine/ medical Intervention: surgical Removal of tumor at the back at the age of 42 years, Uterus Removal at the age of 26, Calcium supplements

Intervention (Diet Therapy): Followed strict DIP diet for 6 months and subsequently followed standard DIP diet.

Outcome: After Two years

Present Status: Complete body healed, slight osteopenia at lower back, now a Marathon Runner

Discomforts: No discomfort except stiffness

Medications: Nil

Life -saving W.I.S.E truth

Nothing less than a miracle from Medical Science point of view, Simi Handa (Pharmacist), with severe osteoporosis (-6), bedridden for several months followed by the diagnosis of cancer; now a marathon runner, a full- time proponent of the DIP DIET and is a part of our W.I.S.E Team.

45

Uterine Fibroid, cysts in ovaries, kidney stones, Low hemoglobin

Medical history of the patient at the time when she contacted us:

Mallareddy Bharati, 42yrs, from Andhra Pradesh, India contacted us on 20 September 2020 through Virtual OPD/VOPD

Diagnosis: Uterine Fibroid, cysts in ovaries, kidney stones, Hb-6.5gm/dl

Discomforts: Lower back pain, knee pain for the last 3 years, currently suffering from severe lower back pain

Medicines/ medical intervention: Nil

Intervention (Diet Therapy): The customized DIP diet plan was followed from 26-Sep-20 for 3 months and subsequently followed standard DIP Diet.

Outcome: After 3 months.

Present Status: Symptomatically no discomfort

Discomforts: Nil

Medications: Nil

Life -saving W.I.S.E truth

Pain in the several places in the body along with kidney stone, cyst in the ovaries and uterine fibroid, just imagine what would have been the fate of the patient had she decided to go for conventional treatment which includes multiple surgery and high dose of lethal medication. Luckily for Mallareddy, just 4 months of DIP Diet could bring her health back on track.

46

Panic attacks, anxiety & gastritis

Medical history of the patient at the time when he contacted us:

Sujan V, 27yrs, from Karnataka, India contacted us on 2 Nov 2020 through Virtual OPD/VOPD

Diagnosis: Condition/case- Severe gastric, breathing tightness when gastric released I will feel relaxed, panic attacks like uncontrolled shivering and unexplained problems, stress and anxiety nerves weakness.

Discomforts: Severe gastritis, feeling tightness while breathing, panic attacks, stress and anxiety, nerve weakness.

Medicines/ medical intervention: Nexito

Intervention (Diet Therapy): The customized DIP diet plan was prescribed on 12-Nov-20 to be followed for 3 months followed by standard DIP Diet after completion of 3 months.

Outcome: After 2 and a half months

Present Status: Much relief, gastric issues cured now, feeling better.

Discomforts: Nil

Medications: Nil

Life -saving W.I.S.E truth

Getting rid of 3 mutually exclusive burden, like severe gastric issues, panic attacks, and deadly antidepressant drug in just 2 and a half months would seem to be an impossible expectation from the conventional doctor's point of view but Sujan could make it possible with DIP Diet.

47

Thyroid, diabetes, High BP & Heart disease

Medical history of the patient at the time when he contacted us:

Vivek Kumar, 57yrs, from Nepal contacted us on 4 April 2020 through Virtual OPD/VOPD

Diagnosis: High BP, Heart disease, thyroid, pain in the joints & bones

Discomforts: Weakness, disturbed sleep, pain in left hip, mild pain in the heart

Medicines/medical intervention: Reclidemr30, Vozucam0, Repace25, Mgonce, Ecosprin, Betaloc, Thyroxine, Vitamin D.

Intervention (Diet Therapy): The customized DIP diet plan was followed from 11-Apr-20 for 3 months and subsequently followed standard DIP Diet.

Outcome: After 8 months

Present Status: All parameters normal for diabetes, High BP, heart & thyroid, latest HBA1c is 6

Discomforts: Nil

Medications: Nil

Life -saving W.I.S.E truth

For most of the patients, with medical condition similar to this Nepal resident, have accepted living rest of the life with all the sufferings, but not for Vivek who contacted us through VOPD. Now after 8 months of being on recommended DIP Diet, he is free from all the medicines and all symptoms whatsoever.

48

COVID-19 Symptoms, dangerously low SpO2 (50%), fever & headache

Medical history of the patient at the time when he contacted us:

Dharmendra Kumar, 41yrs, from U.P., India contacted us through N.I.C.E (Network of Influenza Care Experts) initiative and assigned to N.I.C.E practitioner Shikha Saxena

Diagnosis: SpO2 less than 50% (patient has not undergone COVID-19 test)

Discomforts: Breathlessness, Fever, Headache, Body ache

Medicines/ medical intervention: Nil

Intervention (Diet Therapy): The 3-step flu diet was followed from 09-Oct-20 for 3 days followed by standard DIP Diet till recovery

Outcome: After 7 days

Present Status: completely cured

Discomforts: Nil

Medications: Nil

Life -saving N.I.C.E truth

An SpO2 less than 50% warrants nothing less than a mechanical ventilator and lots of prayer for the Patient's survival, even than almost 100%of such Patients could not survive, but for Dharmendra Kumar, a simple prone ventilation technique (which anyone can learn in 1 minute) and DIP Diet is all that was need to recover completely from otherwise a life-threatening medical condition

49

C0VID-19 Symptoms Dry cough & low SpO_2

Medical history of the patient at the time when he/she contacted us:

Surjit Singh, 63yrs, from Punjab, India contacted us through N.I.C.E (Network of Influenza Care Experts) initiative and assigned to N.I.C.E practitioner Vijay Anand

Diagnosis: Dry Cough, low SpO_2

Discomforts: Breathlessness, Body ache/muscle ache, Tiredness, Weakness.

Medicines/ medical intervention: No

Intervention (Diet Therapy): The customized DIP diet plan was followed from 05-Oct-20 onwards till complete recovery

Outcome: After 7 days

Status: Completely cured

Discomforts: Nil

Medications: Nil

Life -saving N.I.C.E truth:

Our N.I.C.E Expert Vijay Anand handled the case of Surjit Singh who presented himself with dry cough and low SpO_2 level. Customized DIP Diet Protocol and prone ventilation was enough for Surjit to recover within a week

50

COVID-19, Dry Cough & Chest Pain

Medical history of the patient at the time when he contacted us:

Vinesh Hosurkar, 44yrs, from Pune, India contacted us on 25th Sept-20 through N.I.C.E (Network of Influenza Care Experts) initiative and assigned to N.I.C.E practitioner Simmi Handa

Diagnosis: COVID-19

Discomforts: Dry Cough, Chest Pain,

Medicines/ medical intervention: Nil

Intervention (Diet Therapy): The customized 3 step Diet plan was followed from 26 September 20 till completely recovery

Outcome: After 3 days

Status: Completely cured & healthy

Discomforts: Nil

Medications: Nil

Life -saving N.I.C.E truth:

Vinesh Hosurkar a COVID-19 Patient contacted our N.I.C.E. practitioner Simmi Handa, through our official COVID helpline just like our more than 50,000 successfully treated COVID-19 / ILI patient, he got cured with our Flu Diet Protocol.

51

Dry Cough, heart problem, acidity & bloating

Medical history of the patient at the time when he contacted us:

Arvind Tiwari, 33years, from Mumbai, India contacted us on 7 July 2020 through N.I.C.E (Network of Influenza Care Experts) and assigned to our N.I.C.E. practitioner Thokchom Rameshwar Singh.

Diagnosis: Dry cough, Heart Problem, acidity

Discomforts: Breathlessness, Gas, bloating, excessive cough

Medicine/Intervention: Nil.

Intervention (Diet Therapy): The 3 Step Flu diet plan was followed from 7 July 2020 for 3 days and subsequently followed standard DIP Diet till recovery.

Outcome: After 3 months

Present Status: Completely cured all health issues.

Discomforts: Nil

Medications: Nil

Life -saving N.I.C.E truth

Arvind, enrolled in N.I.C.E for dry cough and breathlessness; but was diagnosed with heart problem. He cured his dry cough with 3 Step Flu Diet and decided to directly follow the DIP Diet bypassing the conventional medicine protocol. Within a month not only got complete relief from all the symptoms of heart problem but as a bonus get relief from a lingering stomach issue as well.

52

COVID-19, Loss of taste & smell

Medical history of the patient at the time when he/she contacted us:

Abhishek Vashishtha, 19yrs from Dehradun, India contacted us on 12 July 2020 through N.I.C.E (Network of Influenza Care Experts) and assigned to our N.I.C.E. practitioner Narendra.

Diagnosis: COVID-19

Discomforts: Loss of taste, Loss of smell

Medicine/Intervention: Nil

Intervention (Diet Therapy): The 3 Step Flu diet plan was followed from 12 July 2020 for 3 days and subsequently followed standard DIP Diet for a week.

Outcome: After 2 days

Status: Completely recovered

Discomforts: Nil

Medications: Nil

Life -saving N.I.C.E truth

Abhishek, a Corona positive patient with a classic symptom of loss of taste and smell contacted us through our N.I.C.E network. Our N.I.C. E expert Narender handled the case and guided him with our standard Protocols of DIP Diet. It took just 48 hours to recover from the symptoms.

53

Snoring, Hypertension, Diabetes & High Cholesterol

Medical history of the patient at the time when he contacted us:

Sanjeev Kumar, 49years, from New Delhi, India contacted us after watching YouTube Video

Diagnosis: Hypertension, Diabetes, High Cholesterol, snoring.

D**iscomforts:** High sugar readings, high BP, snoring

Medicine/Intervention: Earlier used to take a lot of medicines for issues mentioned above

Intervention (Diet Therapy): The DIP diet plan was followed through You Tube Videos and continued the diet plan till date.

Outcome: After 1 month of following the DIP Diet

Status: Sugar lies within 250 range, BP normal, feeling energetic.

Discomforts: Nil

Medications: Nil

Life -saving W.I.S.E truth

Hypertension, Diabetes and high Cholesterol medicines all come in a package especially if; you are 40+ and frequently visit a corporate hospital in the name of preventive health checkup. For Sanjeev, it was a no different story until he saw a video of DIP Diet on internet & within the 1st month on DIP Diet, he could free himself all the 3 D's i.e., Diseases, Drugs & Doctors.

54

HIGH FEVER (104^0 to 105^0 F)

Medical history of the patient at the time when he contacted us:

Mehek Joshi, 10 years, from Maharashtra, India contacted us on 7 August 2020 through N.I.C.E (Network of Influenza Care Experts) and assigned to our N.I.C.E. practitioner Suresh Chautalia

Diagnosis: Continuous high fever 104^0 to 105^0 for 5 days.

Discomforts: High Fever, Body Pain, Headache, Severe pain in legs.

Medicine/Intervention: Paracetamol

Intervention (Diet Therapy): The 3 Step Flu diet plan was followed from 7 August 2020 for 3 days and subsequently followed standard DIP Diet till recovery.

Outcome: After 5 days

Status: Completely cured, no pain in legs, no headache, no body pain

Discomforts: Nil

Medications: Nil

Life -saving N.I.C.E truth

While trying to control with Paracetamol, fever as high as 105-degree Fahrenheit can cause anyone to panic, but not for Mehek, who had complete faith on our N.I.C.E Expert and followed the 3-Step Flu Diet and cold compress to safely come out of the flu.

55

Jaundice & Blood in Urine

Medical history of the patient at the time when he contacted us:

Suraj Kumar, 32years, from New Delhi, India followed DIP diet after watching our You Tube Video

Diagnosis: Jaundice with bilirubin 12.3, bleeding in urine.

Discomforts: Bleeding in urine, pain, breathlessness

Medicine/Intervention: Nil

Intervention (Diet Therapy): The DIP diet plan was followed from You Tube Videos

Outcome: After 5 days

Status: Bilirubin reduced from 12.3 to 3.72 within 5 days, bleeding stopped completely

Discomforts: Nil

Medications: Nil

Life -saving W.I.S.E truth:

Bleeding in urine, Jaundice and abnormally high bilirubin are enough reasons to get admitted to ICU but for Suraj Kumar, DIP Diet at the comfort of his home was enough to get rid of all of his medical issues, permanently!

56

Pneumonia & Asthma

Medical history of the patient:

Triveni, 35years, from Hyderabad, India followed DIP diet after watching our You Tube Videos

Diagnosis: Pneumonia, Asthma since childhood

Discomforts: Sweating, Breathlessness, cough, wheezing

Medicine/Intervention: Earlier used to take a lot of medicines but stopped while taking Diet.

Intervention (Diet Therapy): The DIP diet plan was followed from You Tube Videos

Outcome: After 3 months

Present Status: Recovered from pneumonia & asthma completely

Discomforts: Nil

Medications: Nil

Life -saving W.I.S.E truth

For Triveni recovering from childhood Asthma at the age of 35 years, is nothing less than a miracle specially when all available treatment options failed. Just watching a video and getting to know about the DIP Diet and deciding to give it a try, is what led to the dream coming true, that is, for the first time in her life, breathing made easy!

57

Hydrocele, Varicose Veins & Piles

Medical history of the patient :

Shyam Singh, 44years, from UP, India followed DIP diet after watching our YouTube Videos

Diagnosis: Hydrocele, Varicose veins, Piles

Discomforts: Pain, blood in stool.

Medicine/Intervention: Nil

Intervention (Diet Therapy): The DIP diet plan was followed from You Tube Videos

Outcome: After 7 months

Status: Piles and varicose veins completely cured; Hydrocele cured 60 %

Discomforts: 40% hydrocele problem persists

Medications: Nil

Life -saving W.I.S.E truth:

Varicose Veins, a condition which is known to only aggravate with time and age with no hope of recovery, but for Shyam, one video changed his understanding about the body's ability to reverse any medical condition. Understanding the DIP Diet through video and adopting it religiously, helped him reverse the otherwise known to be irreversible medical condition with of course a side benefit; could cure the Piles.

58

Typhoid

Medical history of the patient at the time when he/she contacted us:

Akshata Yashwant, 22years from Mumbai, India contacted us on 29 June 2020 through N.I.C.E (Network of Influenza Care Experts) and was assigned to our N.I.C.E practitioner Saunak Das.

Diagnosis: Typhoid (WIDAL Test Positive)

Discomforts: High Fever (103^0 F), Body ache.

Medicine/Intervention: Nil

Intervention (Diet Therapy): The 3 Step Flu diet plan was followed from 29 June 2020 for 3 days and subsequently followed standard DIP Diet for 14 days.

Outcome: After 3 days

Status: Completely recovered

Discomforts: Nil

Medications: Nil

Life -saving N.I.C.E truth:

The 3 Step Flu Diet could help Akshata to cure Typhoid in 3 days followed by the DIP Diet for 14 days to replenish the lost nutrients due to illness.

59

Covid Positive, High fever, Diabetes, Piles & Hypertension

Medical history of the patient at the time when he/she contacted us:

Deepak Vishwakarma, 62years, from Jagdalpur, India contacted us on 13 September 2020 through N.I.C.E (Network of Influenza and Care Experts) initiative and assigned to N.I.C.E Practitioner

Diagnosis: Diabetes, Hypertension, Piles, Chronic high fever 103 degrees and Spo2 of 92

Discomforts: Very high fever for 10 days, High Blood sugar readings, Blood in stools.

Medicine/medicalintervention: ParacetamolHydroxychloroquine

Intervention (Diet Therapy): The 3 Step Flu Diet was followed from 14 September 2020 for 3 days and subsequently followed standard DIP Diet

Outcome: After 7 days

Present Status: Completely cured his COVID-19 symptoms within 7 days and very happy.

Discomforts: Nil

Medications: Nil

Life -saving N.I.C.E truth:

Deepak presented himself to us with High Fever and low SPO2 with several co-morbid conditions, clearly fit for ICU. Instead, we put him on the 3 step Flu Diet. He recovered from all the symptoms in the comfort of his home.

60

Rheumatoid Arthritis, Thyroid, Diabetes & High Cholesterol

Medical history of the patient:

Archana Jain, 47years, from Surat, India followed DIP diet after watching our YouTube Videos

Diagnosis: Rheumatoid Arthritis, Thyroid (TSH 6.8), High Cholesterol, Diabetes

Discomforts: Acidity, muscle cramps, pain in joints, muscle tightening, muscle pulling.

Medicine/ Intervention: Handful of medicines

Intervention (Diet Therapy): The DIP diet plan was followed from You Tube Videos

Outcome: After 40 Days

Status: Cholesterol, Diabetes normalized, TSH level reduced to 4.02, feeling more energetic, acidity bloating completely cured, symptoms of rheumatoid arthritis substantially reduced, excess weight reduced by 4 kg.

Discomforts: Nil

Medications: Nil

Life -saving W.I.S.E truth/ Analysis:

Bringing back the TSH to 4, reducing weight by 4 kgs and recovery from 4 other mutually exclusive illnesses (Rheumatoid Arthritis, Acidity, Diabetes and Muscle cramp) with just 40 days of DIP Diet. It all started with just watching a video on DIP Diet on internet and ended up with stopping all medications!

61

Motorbike accident with multiple stitches on face few days before wedding

Medical history of the patient at the time when he contacted us:

Manoj Pandey, age 28yrs from U.P had a motorbike accident on 28th Oct,2020 and contacted us on 02 Nov, 2020 through his brother Sanjay Pandey who is a close associate of ours.

Diagnosis: Motor Accident with wounds and stitches all over face and other body parts due to accident

Discomforts: Pain & wounds

Medicine/ medical intervention: Antibiotics and pain killers

Intervention (Diet Therapy): 'Accelerated Wound Healing Diet Protocol' was followed from 02 Nov-20 and subsequently followed customized DIP Diet till recovery.

Outcome: After 22 Days

Present Status: Perfectly cured, no scars on face. Diet started from 02 November 2020, and the wedding took place on 25th Nov 2020.

Discomforts: Nil

Medications: Nil

Life -saving W.I.S.E truth:

To believe, you have to see his video on **www.coronakaal.tv/onequestion**. A motorbike accident a few days before wedding was a nightmare for Manoj Pandey who almost decided to postpone the marriage. As he was 100% certain that all his wounds and scars will take months to heal. But luckily for his brother Sanjay Pandey, just mentioned about him during one of our video shoots in our office. An immediate 'Accelerated Wound Healing Diet Protocol' helped him completely recover from the pain, wounds & stitch marks by the wedding day.

62

Dengue

Medical history of the patient at the time when he contacted us:

Udayveer, age 25yrs from Agra, India contacted our Diabetes Educator Vishal Saini for DIP diet treatment

Diagnosis: Dengue

Discomforts: High fever, body pain, constipation, acidity, hair fall

Medicine/medical intervention: None

Intervention (Diet Therapy): The 3 Step Flu diet plan was followed for 3 Days and subsequently followed standard DIP Diet.

Outcome: After 3 Days

Status: Perfectly healthy

Discomforts: Nil

Medications: Nil

Life -saving N.I.C.E truth:

Just 3 days was enough for Udayveer to cure all the symptoms of Dengue with the 3 step Flu Diet. As a side benefit, could also cure constipation by subsequently following the DIP Diet.

63

Lung Infection & Diabetes

Medical history of the patient at the time when he contacted us:

Mohan Lal Bajaj, 63 years, from Agra, India contacted our Diabetes Educator Vishal Saini in 2019 for DIP diet treatment

Diagnosis: Lung Infection, Diabetes,

Discomforts: High Blood Sugar readings, breathlessness

Medicine/Intervention: 10-15 medicines.

Intervention (Diet Therapy): The customized DIP diet plan was followed for 3 months and subsequently followed standard DIP Diet till now.

Outcome: After 3 months

Status: Now perfectly fine, Stopped all the medicines, very much satisfied and happy.

Discomforts: Nil

Medications: Nil

Life -saving W.I.S.E truth:

A customized DIP Diet and a few months of patience is all that was needed for Mohan Lal to cure two mutually exclusive medical conditions and escape about a dozen of pills.

64

Hernia & Hypertension

Medical history of the patient at the time when she contacted us:

Parimala, 54 yrs, from Bangalore contacted our Diabetes Educator Vishal Saini in 2019 for DIP diet treatment

Diagnosis: Hernia, Hypertension

Discomforts: Continuously increasing blood pressure readings, pain in hernial site (surgery suggested)

Medicine/Intervention: BP medicines dosage increased from 20 mg to 60 mg within 5 years

Intervention (Diet Therapy): The DIP diet plan was followed from 2019 onwards.

Outcome: After 3 months

Present Status: No Surgery required for Hernia, perfectly fine. BP readings normal.

Discomforts: Nil

Medications: Nil

Life -saving W.I.S.E truth:

For most of the patients, an increase in the dosage of B.P. medication is often geometric progression. For Parimala, she could not only halt this steady ever-increasing dose of medication but could also get rid of the medicine by adopting the DIP Diet.

65

Bone Tuberculosis, 80 % Liver Damage, Depression & Hyperacidity

Medical history of the patient:

Jitendra Srivastava, 67 years, from Madhya Pradesh contacted Mr Ashok from Wholesome Tales

Diagnosis: Bone TB, 80 % Liver Damage, Hyperacidity, Depression

Discomforts: Pain, acidity, Depression, backbone was bent at 90 degrees, could not eat anything

Medicine/Intervention: Had taken a lot of medicines

Intervention (Diet Therapy): The customized DIP diet plan was followed for 3 months and subsequently followed standard DIP Diet.

Outcome: After 3 months

Status: Cured Bone TB, Liver is working fine, recovered from depression, No pain

Discomforts: Nil

Medications: Nil

Life -saving W.I.S.E truth:

Uncountable pills and unimaginable pain as a result of a 90-degree bend in the backbone was a few of the things, Jitendra Srivastava was dealing with until he started the DIP Diet. Now with zero medicine and zero discomfort, life back on track, is nothing less than a miracle. With the modern health care system all this would not have been possible even remotely.

66

Jaundice

Medical history of the patient at the time when he contacted us:

Abhnam Aggrawal, 4.5 years, from UP, India contacted us through N.I.C.E and was assigned to our N.I.C.E practitioner Ravi Biswas

Diagnosis: Jaundice

Discomforts: Whole body became pale, mustard oil colored urine, loss of appetite, loss of physical activities, lethargic all the time

Medicine/ medical intervention: Nil

Intervention (Diet Therapy): The 3 Step Flu Diet plan was followed for 3 days and subsequently followed standard DIP Diet

Outcome: After 15 Days

Status: Jaundice cured, appetite increased, now he is active.

Discomforts: Nil

Medications: Nil

Life -saving N.I.C.E truth:

A 3 Step Flu Diet for 3 days followed by the DIP Diet was enough for the 4.5-year-old boy to recover from Jaundice. No Medication was given in the whole process of recovery.

67

PCOD, Fatty Liver & Obesity

Medical history of the patient:

Veenu, 34years, from India contacted our Diabetes Educator Gayatree Arya on 18th Aug,2020

Diagnosis: Fatty liver, PCOD, overweight, high pus cells found in CBC report

Discomforts: Loss of energy, weight issues

Medicine/Intervention: Earlier used to take 3-4 medicines.

Intervention (Diet Therapy): The DIP diet plan recommended by Gayatree Arya was followed for 3 months

Outcome: After 3 months

Status: Cured PCOD, Fatty liver &reduced weight from 76 kg to 69kg

Discomforts: Nil

Medications: Nil

Life -saving W.I.S.E truth:

Three mutually exclusive medical conditions (fatty liver, PCOD and obesity) and 3 pills, this is all she could get rid-of within 3 months of following the DIP Diet. However, she decided to follow the Dip Diet protocol lifelong to avoid any future illness!

68

Trigeminal Neuralgia

Medical history of the patient:

Sanjay Kumar from Ujjain contacted Mr Ashok of Wholesome Tales Youtube Channel

Diagnosis: Trigeminal Neuralgia

Discomforts: Severe Pain

Medicine/Intervention: Used to take Pain killers for trigeminal neuralgia

Intervention (Diet Therapy): The DIP diet plan was followed till complete recovery

Outcome: As per video testimonial

Present Status: Cured neuralgia & hypertension

Discomforts: Nil

Medications: Nil

Life -saving W.I.S.E truth:

Trigeminal Neuralgia, a medical condition infamous for striking many celebrities (Salman Khan, Asharam Bapu) and known to be an incurable painful disease. However, for Sanjay Kumar, watching a YouTube channel 'Wholesome Tales' changed his life. He learned about the DIP Diet through the video and could cure the incurable within a few months of following the diet. As a side benefit, he could overcome hypertension as well.

69

Chronic Constipation & Hyperacidity

Medical history of the patient:

Megha, 25years, from Chandigarh contacted our Diabetes Educator Vishal Saini in 2019

Diagnosis: Chronic constipation, Hyperacidity Since many years

Discomforts: Acidity, constipation, low energy levels.

Medicine/ medical intervention: Used to take many medicines for acidity and constipation for many years.

Intervention (Diet Therapy): The DIP diet plan was recommended by Vishal Saini.

Outcome: As per testimonial given by the patient

Present Status: Feeling perfectly fine, no more acidity and constipation, energy levels improved

Discomforts: Nil

Medications: Stopped all the medicines

Life -saving W.I.S.E truth:

In urban India chronic constipation has become one of the major medical conditions for many, with which they live permanently assuming that it does not have any cure. For Megha, the story is no different till she met our Diabetes Educator Vishal Saini. Now she is free from all the symptoms and discomfort whatsoever and is leading a great life with DIP diet minus all pills.

70

Plantar Fascitis

Medical history of the patient at the time when she contacted us:

Priyanka Chandra, 30years, from Telangana, India contacted us on 28 April 2020 through Virtual OPD

Diagnosis: Pain in plantar fascia-heel due to Inflammation

Discomforts: Pain in both heels even with touch & while walking.

Medicine/ medical intervention: Elbion PB, Loycoral Plus, Synertab, ACB Plus

Intervention (Diet Therapy): The customized DIP diet plan was followed from 30 April 2020 for 3 months and subsequently followed standard DIP Diet.

Outcome: After 3 months

Present Status: Very much relief, weight loss, feeling energetic.

Discomforts: Nil

Medications: Nil

Life -saving W.I.S.E truth

There is no medicine for treating plantar fascitis and often remains a lifelong suffering which sometimes progresses rapidly. However Priyanka Chandra could get rid of it with the DIP Diet.

71

Piles, Diabetes & Fatty Liver

Medical history of the patient at the time when she contacted us:

Supriya Rana, 44 years, from West Bengal contacted us on 9 August 2019 through 72 Hours Virtual Diabetes Reversal Program.

Diagnosis: Piles, Fatty Liver, Diabetes

Discomforts: Itchiness, weakness, acidity, dizziness

Medicine/ medical intervention: No medications

Intervention (Diet Therapy): The customized diet plan was followed from 9 August 2019 for 3 days and subsequently followed standard DIP Diet till recovery.

Outcome: After 3 months

Present Status: Complete recovery from piles, fatty liver, acidity and diabetes

Discomforts: Nil

Medications: Nil

Life -saving W.I.S.E truth:

With 4 mutually exclusive medical conditions and a handful of medicines, Supriya contacted us with the hope of a cure. Now at the time of the book going to the press, she is living a disease-free & medicine-free life while being on a DIP Diet.

72

Diabetes & Hypertension

Medical history of the patient at the time when she contacted us:

Saida khatoon, 57 years, from Bihar, India contacted us on 8 September 2020 through Virtual OPD

Diagnosis: Diabetes, Blood pressure

Discomforts: Loss of Appetite, Insomnia, Shoulder Pain, Burning Sensation in Left foot, Knee Pain, Dizziness.

Medicine/Intervention: Methobact, Fenocar 20, Etorag 90, Animefix Beta, Valera, Flurag 20

Intervention (Diet Therapy): The customized DIP diet plan was followed from 10 September 2020 for 3 months and subsequently followed standard DIP Diet.

Outcome: After 3 months

Present Status: Diabetes and blood pressure in healthy range as per patient's feelings, energetic and fine.

Discomforts: Nil

Medications: Sometimes Pain killer for Knee Pain.

Life -saving W.I.S.E truth:

After suffering from multiple disorders for more than a decade and with a long list of discomfort and cocktail, now with DIP Diet all symptoms gone and also free from most of the drugs.

73

Cerebral atrophy & Diabetes Type 2

Medical History of the patient:

Nathu Ram Mangla, Age: 62 years from New Delhi came in contact with our Diabetes Educator Amrita Jain in December 2020.

Diagnosis: Cerebral atrophy, Diabetes type 2

Discomforts: Bedridden with loss of memory for one whole year, incoherent speech, verge of going into coma

Medicine/ medical Intervention: Tablet Volix Trio, Tablet Vilact, Ecosprin, Tablet Neferosave,Tablet D3 Must, Tablet Mega Cartigen, Pregabid NT tablet, Tablet Urineax,Tablet Fuicon

Intervention (Diet Therapy): Followed Customized DIP diet from 1st December 2020

Outcome: within 1.5 months at the time of printing of this book

Present Status: He is able to talk, walk properly and has started going to office along with his son.

Discomforts: Nothing except excess urination

Medications: Tablet Vilact

Life -saving W.I.S.E truth:

Nathu Ram Mangla was on the verge of a coma when his family members contacted our Diabetes Educator, Amrita Jain. Now he is able to speak, comprehend and walk and has also joined the office along with his son . To believe this, watch his testimonial video at www.coronakaal.tv/onequestion.

74

Tuberculosis & COVID Positive twice in a month

Medical history of the patient at the time when he contacted us:

Bhakti Ratan Vijay, 72 years, from Rajasthan, India contacted us on 24 September 2020 through N.I.C.E and was assigned to our N.I.C.E practitioner Amarnath V Gaonkar

Diagnosis: Tuberculosis and Tested COVID Positive twice in one month

Discomforts: Fever, Cough, Congestion, Tiredness, Weakness and Body ache

Medicine/ medical intervention: Paracetamol, erythromycin for TB

Intervention (Diet Therapy): The 3 Step Flu diet was followed for 3 days from 25 September 2020 onwards and subsequently followed standard DIP Diet.

Outcome: After 10 days as per video testimonial

Present Status: Completely Cured

Discomforts: Nil

Medications: Nil

Life -saving N.I.C.E truth:

Patient with COVID -19 and with tuberculosis as a pre-existing condition may appear to be a scary situation to many. However, just by adopting the 3 Step Flu Diet followed by DIP Diet, it was a smooth and rapid journey to recovery for Bhakti Ratan Vijay in the comfort of his home.

75

Morbid Obesity

Medical history of the patient:

Vidya Agar, 57years, from Gurugram, India contacted our Diabetes Educator Rashmi Jain in June 2019

Diagnosis: Morbidly Obese (weight 142 kgs)

Discomforts: Weight issues like, breathlessness, body pain, legs pain

Medicine/ medical intervention: Nil

Intervention (Diet Therapy): The DIP diet plan was followed from 20 June 2019 and being followed till date

Outcome: As per video testimonial

Present Status: Current weight:124 Kg lost 18 kgs weight within 3 months by following only 60-70% diet. Now want to follow 100% diet to reduce more 30 kgs weight, highly motivated, feeling good and perfectly fine.

Discomforts: Nil

Medications: Nil

Life -saving W.I.S.E truth

Partially following the dip diet, Vidya Agar was relieved off the pain and breathlessness and as a side benefit also reduced 18 kg weight. Our Diabetes Educator Rashmi Jain helped her to overcome the illness.

76

Fibromyalgia & PCOD

Medical history of the patient :

Sneha Acharya, 37 years, from Mumbai, India contacted our Diabetes Educator Rashmi Jain in June 2019

Diagnosis: Fibromyalgia PCOD.

Discomforts: Very painful, sometimes bedridden due to the extreme pain in all the muscles of the body.

Medicine/ medical intervention: Nerve smoothness and muscle relaxants.

Intervention (Diet Therapy): The DIP diet plan was followed from June 2018 onwards

Outcome: As per video testimonial

Present Status: Fibromyalgia completely cured, no more pain, PCOD cured as conceived normally, throughout pregnancy was normal at the age of 37 years

Discomforts: Nil.

Medications: Nil

Life -saving W.I.S.E truth:

After failing all kinds of treatment and remaining painfully bedridden for months, Sneha finally got in touch with our Diabetes Educator Rashmi Jain and could free herself of two mutually exclusive life-threatening illnesses, with just one diet, namely the DIP Diet.

77

Diabetes, Hypertension & Obesity

Medical history of the patient:

Hardeep Kumar Mahajan, 64 years, from Faridabad, India contacted Rashmi Jain in March 2018

Diagnosis: Diabetes, Hypertension, obesity

Discomforts: High sugar readings, High BP readings, weight 102kg.

Medicine/ medical intervention: 80 units insulin/day along with two more medicines

Intervention (Diet Therapy): The customized DIP diet plan was followed from march 2018 and subsequently followed standard DIP Diet.

Outcome: As per video testimonial

Present Status: Insulin free, BP is normal, lost 16 kg weight in 2 months., current weight 86 kg.

Discomforts: Nil

Medications: Nil

Life -saving W.I.S.E truth:

Heavily dependent on Insulin, the morbidly obese Hardeep Mahajan is a well reputed businessman of Faridabad. He shocked his friends when he lost 16 Kgs of weight and also got rid of Insulin totally within a few weeks of meeting our Diabetes educator Rashmi Jain. He modified the DIP Diet so as to satisfy his taste buds and now spends substantial time educating people on using food as medicine.

Diabetes Type 1

Medical history of the patient at the time when his parents contacted us:

Achint (name changed), 8 years contacted us in August 2018 through 72 hrs. Diabetes Reversal Virtual Tour

Diagnosis: Diabetes Type 1

Discomforts: Low energy, very weak

Medicine/Intervention: 12 units Insulin /day

Intervention (Diet Therapy): The customized DIP diet plan was followed from August 2018 and subsequently followed standard DIP Diet.

Outcome: At the time of print of this book

Present Status: Reduced dose of insulin- taking 1 unit 3 times.

Discomforts: Good energy level, immunity got stronger

Medications: 3 units/day

Life -saving W.I.S.E truth

A Diabetes Type 1 Child, was taking 12 units insulin at the time, when he contacted us. Now by following DIP Diet, he could reduce dependency on Insulin by ¾th and taking just 3 units/day. Hopefully stricter adherence to the diet and sunlight will help him to be totally insulin free.

79

Triple Vessel Disease

Medical history of the patient at the time when he contacted us:

Vijay Kumar, 46years, from Punjab contacted us on 23 October 2020 through Virtual OPD

Diagnosis: Triple vessel disease, heart attack on 8 /10/2020 and stenting done.

Discomforts: Chest Pain, discomfort while climbing stairs, Breathlessness.

Medicine/ Medical intervention: Nitrocontin, Ramipril, Carca, Brilinta, Ecosprin, Atorvas

Intervention (Diet Therapy): The customized DIP diet plan was recommended from 25 October 2020 for 3 months and subsequently standard DIP Diet to be followed.

Outcome: After 2 months

Present Status: Feeling Good

Discomforts: Mild discomfort when climbing stairs.

Medications: Nil

Life -saving W.I.S.E truth

Even after multiple stenting, Vijay could not get relief, he contacted us. Now after 2 months of following the prescribed DIP diet, he is free of all medicines and the symptoms reduced drastically.

80

Autism & Diabetes Type 1

Medical history of the patient at the time when his parents contacted us:

Gaurav Gupta, 12years, from New Delhi contacted us on 26 May 2020 through Virtual OPD/VOPD

Diagnosis: Diabetes Type 1 with Autism

Discomforts: High Blood sugar readings, No proper sleep at night, problem in comprehending things, learning difficulties.

Medicine/ medical intervention: Insulin- Wosulin 30/7 (5 unit), Lantus 3- 4 units/day, Sugar tom 20ml, Tab.Pioglitazone.

Intervention (Diet Therapy): The customized DIP diet plan was followed from 22 June 2020 and subsequently followed standard DIP Diet.

Outcome: After 3 months

Present Status: Great improvement, Now Listening and understanding things,

Discomforts: Nil

Medications: Insulin Lantus 4 units in a day.

Life -saving W.I.S.E truth

Once a rare and unheard disease, now Autism and Diabetes type 1 is becoming more and more common, more so as a result of ever-increasing number of vaccinations among children. Gaurav could overcome the symptoms of autism to a great extent with the help of the recommended DIP Diet and also minimizing the dependency on insulin/medicine.

81

Psoriasis, Fatty Liver, Severe Acidity & Insomnia

Medical history of the patient:

Ritu Goenka 54 years, contacted our Diabetes Educator Sunita Arya in February 2019

Diagnosis: Constipation, Obesity, Fatty Liver, BP, Psoriasis, Severe Acidity, Sleep problem

Discomforts: Insomnia, skin rashes, overweight.

Medicine/ medical intervention: Restyl 0.25

Intervention (Diet Therapy): The customized DIP diet plan was followed from February 2019 onwards till the time of making the video testimonial

Outcome: As per Video Testimonial

Status: Totally reversed fatty liver, acidity, constipation, great Relief in Psoriasis (80-90%), obesity- lost 22 kgs weight, normal BP and sleep is normal.

Discomforts: Nil

Medications: Nil

Life -saving W.I.S.E truth:

Ritu Goenka was suffering from 7 seemingly mutually exclusive medical conditions until she met our Diabetes Educator Sunita Arya. With a customised DIP diet as advised by Sunita, she recovered from most of those listed health issues.

82

Crohn's Disease

Medical history of the patient:

Manish Agrawal, 44yrs, from Birmingham, United Kingdom contacted our Nutrition Therapist Meena Gupta in January 2020

Diagnosis: Crohn's Disease diagnosed in March 2019, polyps on colonoscopy

Discomforts: Pain in stomach, motions multiple times

Medicine/Intervention: Steroids, mesalazine- Pentasa, Azathioprine, proposed -Mercaptopurine

Intervention (Diet Therapy): The customized DIP diet plan was followed from January 2020 for 3 months and subsequently followed standard DIP Diet

Outcome: As per Video Testimonial

Present Status: No pain, stool is ok & well formed.

Discomforts: Nil

Medications: Nil

Life -saving W.I.S.E truth:

Crohn's disease is kept in the category of the list of incurable diseases. But for Manish Aggarwal recovery came after he got the DIP diet protocol from our Nutrition Therapist Meena Gupta.

83

Suicidal thoughts, Arthritis, Diabetes, Hypertension & Anxiety

Medical history of the patient at the time when he contacted us:

Hazari Singh, 67years contacted us in 2018 through VOPD

Diagnosis: Arthritis, Diabetes, Hypertension, anxiety, obesity.

Discomforts: Suicidal thoughts, pain in body & bones, , High Blood Sugar, High Blood pressure.

Medicine/ medical intervention: Metformin, galvus met, shelcal, alprax, nexito, lonogelpan

Intervention (Diet Therapy): The customized DIP diet plan was followed from 2018 for 3 months and subsequently followed standard DIP Diet

Outcome: At the time of print of this book

Status: No pain, diabetes in normal range, blood Pressure is stable, no anxiety, depression gone, now a 'Social Activist'.

Discomforts: Nil

Medications: Nil

Life -saving W.I.S.E truth:

Owner of a 24- hour Chemist Shop in Delhi, he had been on multiple medications for more than 2 decades. He dropped all the medicines in the dustbin on the day of starting the DIP Diet. It has been 2 years since he has been medicine free and disease free as well. Now he spends most of his time spreading awareness about food as medicine.

84

Brain Tumor

Medical history of the patient at the time when he contacted us:

Anil Kumar 51, years, from Noida contacted us in 2012 for personal consultation

Diagnosis: Brain Tumor

Discomforts: No discomforts as such

Medicine/ medical intervention: Never took medicines, directly started following DIP Diet.

Intervention (Diet Therapy): The customized DIP diet plan was followed from 2012 for 3 months and subsequently followed standard DIP Diet

Outcome: At the time of publishing this book

Present Status: Perfectly Fine, Tumor size shrinked

Discomforts: Nil

Medications: Nil

Life -saving W.I.S.E truth:

Diagnosed with brain tumor and almost heading for surgery as advised by the doctor at AIIMS, he met us for a second opinion. Thereafter, he cancelled the surgery and followed DIP diet along with wheatgrass juice. It has been over a decade now, he is absolutely perfect with no discomfort, whatsoever.

85

Blood Cancer

Medical history of the patient at the time when he contacted us:

Praveen Kumar, age 32 years from Panipat, contacted us on 29 October 2014 for personal consultation.

Diagnosis: Blood Cancer with TLC count 2,94,000/ml on 29 October 2014

Discomforts: Pain in left side of abdomen, felt hard lump under heart

Medicine/medical intervention: Imatinib tab

Intervention (Diet Therapy): The customized DIP diet plan was followed from 30 October 2014 till complete recovery

Outcome: As on 5th June -2015

Status: Perfectly Fit and Fine TLC COUNT: 7500, Hb:13.7

Discomforts: Nil

Medications: Nil

Life -saving W.I.S.E truth:

Blood cancer is known for very poor survival rate and a lot of suffering. However for Praveen Kumar, the things changed when he rejected conventional therapy and adopt the DIP diet. Now it has been more than 5 years since he is cancer -free and most of his time is spent in propagating the DIP Diet based therapy.

86

HIV Positive

Medical history of the patient at the time when she contacted us:

Divya Kamlajan 26 years, she was diagnosed with HIV positive in 2016 by NACO and MSACS. She contacted us on 18 June 2018 through our free HIV AIDS helpline.

Diagnosis: HIV POSITIVE

Discomforts: Dizziness, Severe Hair Loss, Weakness, Severe Headache sometimes, Indigestion.

Medicine/ medical intervention: Taking ART Drugs since 21 June 2016 (Efavirenz 600mg, Lamivudine 300 mg, Tenofovir Disoproxil fumarate 300 mg)

Intervention (Diet Therapy): The customized HIV DIP diet plan was followed from 18 June 2018 till complete recovery

Outcome: As on 20th Nov-2019 after 17 months

Present Status: HIV Negative

Discomforts: Nil

Medications: Nil

Life -saving W.I.S.E truth:

Divya is one of the more than 1000 success stories, who were put on the medication for HIV -AIDS. She came in contact with us through our Free HIV - AIDS Helpline and since then stopped all her medicines while following the DIP Diet. Now she is free of all symptoms & discomfort whatsoever. Even more interesting is that she tested negative for HIV-AIDS!

87

Systemic Lupus Erythematosus

Medical history of the patient at the time when she contacted us:

Seema pal, contacted us on 4 April 2020.

Diagnosis: SLE/Systemic lupus erythematosus

Discomforts: skin rashes, weight loss,

Medicine/medical intervention: MMF 500, MP 40, Ramipril, Colecalciferol, Pantoprazole, Acenocoumarol, Torsemide, Paracetamol.

Intervention (Diet Therapy): The customized DIP diet plan was followed only 50 % from 6 April 2020 and subsequently followed standard DIP Diet after 3 months.

Outcome: After 3 Months

Present Status: Weight gained, skin got better, feeling better.

Discomforts: Nil

Medications: MMF 500, Ramiprill

Life -saving W.I.S.E truth:

SLE, a type of inflammatory disease as a result of autoimmune response of the body, known to have no cure but for Seema Pal, luckily, the cure came in the form of DIP Diet. Following the DIP Diet protocol just 50%, she achieved most of her health objectives including much needed weight gain.

88

Throat Carcinoma, Heart disease, diabetes

Medical history of the patient at the time when he contacted us:

Dr Harish Sharma, 66 years contacted us in September 2017 through Personal Consultation

Diagnosis: Throat Carcinoma, Heart disease, diabetes

Discomforts: voice completely gone, high blood sugar readings up to 480 leg pain, difficulty in breathing, backache, suffocation

Medicine/ medical Intervention: 32 radiation therapies, Insulin 40 units /day, Ecosprin, diamicron, along with many more medicines

Intervention (Diet Therapy): The customized DIP diet plan was followed from September 2017 for 3 months and subsequently followed standard DIP Diet

Outcome: At the time of publication of this book

Present Status: voice returned, No medication, completely free from cancer, sugar readings normal, no heart issues

Discomforts: Nil

Medications: Nil

Life -saving W.I.S.E truth:

Dr Harish Sharma (MD), running his own hospital, is among the very few people who has dared heart diseases and bypass surgery followed up with cancer and radiotherapy, leading to diabetes and lifelong insulin dependency. He was at the edge of his life with the burden of countless medications and unbearable pain and discomfort.After trying all possible therapies under the sun, he decided to try the DIP diet. To his surprise it took 4 months to be completely free from medicine /insulin, discomfort & pain.. Now it has been more than 3.5 years since he is living a medicine free and disease-free life, with about 20 km walk daily as a part of his lifestyle.

89

Atrial Septal Defect, Pulmonary Hypertension & Thyroid

Medical history of the patient at the time when he contacted us:

Suresh Chand Sharma, 61years, from Rajasthan contacted us on June 2019 for personal consultation

Diagnosis: Atrial Septal Defect- ASD, arrhythmia, thyroid, pulmonary hypertension. SPO2- 75

Discomforts: Low oxygen level (on oxygen cylinder), difficulty in climbing staircase, gastric issues.

Medicine/ medical intervention: Bosentan 62.5mg, Thyrox 25mg, Alprax, Cyrad, Deriphyllin

Intervention (Diet Therapy): The customized DIP diet plan was followed from June 2019 and subsequently followed standard DIP Diet.

Outcome: After 3 months

Present Status: Normal oxygen level, ASD reduced to 18 from 20, pulmonary hypertension 60 mmHg, no constipation & gastric issues, thyroid normal

Discomforts: Nil.

Medications: Nil.

Life -saving W.I.S.E truth:

Suresh Chandra Sharma lost his job because of the congenital disease (ASD) and continuous dependence on oxygen cylinder. Finding hope in the DIP diet, he could not only get rid of the dependency on oxygen cylinder but could also reverse the disease clinically.

90

PCOD

Medical history of the patient at the time when she contacted us:

Suhavi Jain, 14 years, from New Delhi contacted us on 27 November 2020 through W.I.S.E (Wellness & Inflammatory Care Experts) initiative and was assigned to W.I.S.E expert Hema Singh

Diagnosis: PCOD

Discomforts: Heavy bleeding for entire one month.

Medicine/ medical intervention: Crina -NCR10mg

Intervention (Diet Therapy): The customized 3 Week's W.I.S.E Protocol was followed from 1st December 2020 for 3 weeks and subsequently followed standard DIP Diet.

Outcome: After 3 weeks

Present Status: Bleeding stopped within 3 days and next periods were regular

Discomforts: Nil

Medications: Nil.

Life -saving W.I.S.E truth:

PCOD often leads to brutal & unscientific hysterectomy, in the conventional world but for Suhavi it was a smooth reversal of the disease just by adopting the DIP diet. Now she is free of medicine and also has a regular menstruation cycle.

91

Ulcerative Colitis

Medical history of the patient :

Rohit Soni, 25 years, from Mumbai contacted TV actress Shalu Soni who follows and promotes DIP Diet

Diagnosis: Ulcerative colitis with CRP -77mg/L & Hemoglobin-9

Discomforts: Severe Stomach Pain, Bleeding Stools, Loose Motions ,45 kg weight loss, Gastric Issues, Hemoglobin deficiency, Vitamin B12 deficiency.

Medicine/medical intervention: Used to take a lot of allopathic medicines

Intervention (Diet Therapy): The DIP diet plan was followed from 22 April 2019 onwards

Outcome: As per video testimonial after 8 months

Present Status: CRP-2mg/L, Hb-12.6, no stomach Pain, no bleeding in stools, energy levels are good.

Discomforts: Nil

Medications: Nil

Life -saving W.I.S.E truth:

After trying all possible treatments, he finally decided to be on a DIP diet. In 8 months, he could free himself of the disease symptomatically and also clinically.

92

Bronchial Asthma

Medical history of the patient:

Aaheli Bhattacharya, 15 years, from Kolkata contacted our Nutrition Therapist Meena Gupta in June 2019

Diagnosis: Acute Asthma since childhood

Discomforts: Breathlessness, uncontrollable cough especially during night.

Medicine/ medical intervention: Steroids

Intervention (Diet Therapy): The customized DIP diet plan was followed from June 2019 and subsequently followed standard DIP Diet after 3 months.

Outcome: As per Video Testimonial

Present Status: Asthma has been 90% cured, relief in chest and congestion, cured coughing completely.

Discomforts: Nil

Medications: Nil

Life -saving W.I.S.E truth:

A lifelong disease, ever increasing discomfort and dangerous steroids, Aaheli was going through all this till she decided to be on a DIP Diet. Now free of all symptoms and medication. After trying all possible treatments, she finally decided to be on a DIP Diet. In 8 months, she could free herself of the disease symptomatically and clinically as well.

Diabetes Type 1

Medical history of the patient at the time when he/she contacted us:

Vaibhav (name changed), 11 years, from Bharuch, Gujrat contacted us on Dec 2018 through 72 hrs Virtual Tour.

Diagnosis: Diabetes Type1

Discomforts: High blood sugar readings, weight loss.

Medicine/Intervention: 28 units insulin (Apidra, lantus)4 times a day.

Intervention (Diet Therapy): The customized DIP diet plan was followed from December 2018 for 3 days and subsequently followed the DIP Diet plan 60% only

Outcome: After 3 months

Present Status: energetic, capable of doing abundance of physical activities like Surya namaskar, breathing exercises.

Discomforts: None

Medications: Lantus 5-6 units occasionally in 3-4 days if needed.

Life -saving W.I.S.E truth:

As reported by the parents, the child is following the DIP Diet only upto 60%. Understandably the partial recovery happened from high doses of 2 types of Insulin 4 times a day to small doses of insulin once every 2nd or 3rd day. 'No need to inject insulin every day' is a great hope that the present condition can be improved by encouraging the child to follow the DIP diet more sincerely.

94

Coeliac & Diabetes Type 1

Medical history of the patient at the time when she contacted us:

Surabhi (name changed), 3.8 years, from London, UK contacted us on 20th November 2020 through VOPD

Diagnosis: Diabetes type 1 with Hba1c-12.5mmol/13.6%, coeliac positive

Discomforts: Frequent hunger, weight loss, high blood sugar readings.

Medicine/ medical intervention: Novorapid 1U/ 3times a day + Absaglar penfill -3U

Intervention (Diet Therapy): The customized DIP diet plan was followed from 28 November 2020

Outcome: After 1 month

Present Status: energetic & happy, readings are stabilized HbA1c-6.2%

Discomforts: Nil.

Medications: Nil

Life -saving W.I.S.E truth:

Zero insulin dependency on the day of starting the DIP Diet in case of a Diabetes Type 1 toddler is not only beyond the conceivable imagination of the medical establishment but also a threat to the profit -minded diabetes industry. The case is a living proof that the insulin industry can become absolute if every doctor decides to prescribe the DIP Diet instead of insulin, the moment they come across someone with high blood sugar.

95

Diabetes Type 1

Medical history of the patient:

Sambarta Chakraborty, 15yrs, from Kolkata contacted Nutrition Therapist Meena Gupta on 1st April 2019

Diagnosis: Diabetes Type1, HbA1c 12.25 (29/03/2019), C-peptide-0.463ng/ml

Discomforts: Weight Loss, High blood sugar readings.

Medicine/medical intervention: 15-25 units Insulin in a day.

Intervention (Diet Therapy): The customized DIP diet plan was followed from 5 April 2019 and subsequently followed standard DIP Diet after 3 months.

Outcome: As per video testimonial

Status: Within 10 days, blood sugar readings came normal, now insulin free for more than a year.

Discomforts: Nil.

Medications: Nil

Life -saving W.I.S.E truth:

A Diabetes Type 1 child, Sambarta was told that he will always remain dependent on insulin. He, however, did not accept the conventional wisdom and contacted Meena Gupta. The miracle happened. Within 10 days of following the customized DIP Diet, he was insulin free and had successfully cured diabetes Type 1

96

Fundal Erosion

Medical history of the patient at the time when he contacted us:

Mahadev Sahoo, 33yrs, from Orissa contacted us on 2 December 2020 through W.I.S.E (Wellness and Inflammatory Syndrome Experts) and assigned to expert Hema Singh.

Diagnosis: Fundal Erosion, BP- 190/137, W.B.C - 22000/cumm, eosinophils - 33%

Discomforts: Severe Stomach Pain after Meals, Acidity, Bloating, Constipation.

Medicine/medical intervention: Sompraz 40, Sompraz L, Sucral O, Montek LC, Bandy Plus 12.

Intervention (Diet Therapy): The customized 3 Weeks' W.I.S.E protocol was followed from 5 December 2020 for 3 weeks and subsequently followed standard DIP Diet.

Outcome: After 15 days

Present Status: BP-140/90, WBC-12000/cumm, eosinophils-20%, feeling good now, no stomach pain, no constipation, no acidity and bloating. now, feeling very light.

Discomforts: Nil

Medications: Nil

Life -saving W.I.S.E truth:

The disease if persisted for a long period might get converted into cancer. However, in case of Mahadev, just 15 days on customized DIP diet was enough to symptomatically and clinically cure the disease and escape the unnecessary medicines as well.

97

Recurrent Allergies & Asthma

Medical history of the patient at the time when she contacted us:

Neha Soni 37 yrs. from Kolkata contacted us on 2 December 2020 through W.I.S.E (Wellness and inflammatory syndrome Expert) and assigned to Expert Shabnam Khairdi.

Diagnosis: Asthma, Allergies, Cold, Cough, Sneezing.

Discomforts: Allergies, Breathlessness, Cold, Cough, Sneezing.

Medicine/Intervention: Inhaler Foracort200.

Intervention (Diet Therapy): The customized 3 Weeks' W.I.S.E protocol was followed from 2 December 2020 for 3 Weeks and subsequently standard DIP Diet to be followed.

Outcome: After 3 weeks

Present Status: Asthma along with other allergies have been cured within 3 weeks.

Discomforts: Nil

Medications: Nil

Life -saving W.I.S.E truth:

Otherwise known to be a life long suffering, Neha Soni not only got rid of her recurring allergies & chronic asthma but also her inhaler within just 3 weeks of following the DIP diet.

98

Chronic Kidney Disease with Dialysis & Diabetes

Medical history of the patient:

Bajrang Lal Mittal, 67 yrs, from Kolkata contacted our Diabetes Educator & Nutrition Therapist Meena Gupta on 10 Oct 2019

Diagnosis: Chronic kidney disease with dialysis, diabetes.

Discomforts: Creatinine 7-8

Medicine/medical intervention: weekly dialysis along with other medications.

Intervention (Diet Therapy): The customized DIP diet plan was followed from 16 October 2019 onwards

Outcome: After 10 days of following the diet

Status: Dialysis stopped, creatinine 2.28.

Discomforts: Nil

Medications: Nil

Life -saving W.I.S.E truth:

Dialysis patient Mr Bajrang Lal Mittal with creatinine 7-8 contacted Meena Gupta in October 2019. Soon after starting the prescribed DIP Diet, he got rid of Dialysis permanently. Presently, his creatinine level has reduced to 2.28.

99

Pancreatic Lithiasis & Colitis

Medical history of the patient:

Devansh Agrawal, 16 years, from Darjeeling contacted our Diabetes Educator & Nutrition Therapist Meena Gupta in March 2020.

Diagnosis: Calcification in Pancreas, colitis.

Discomforts: severe stomach ache, gastric issues.

Medicine/ medical intervention: Lupase 25000.

Intervention (Diet Therapy): The Customized DIP diet plan was followed from March 2020 onwards.

Outcome: After 2.5 months

Present Status: No stomach ache, healthy.

Discomforts: Nil

Medications: Nil

Life -saving W.I.S.E truth:

Calcification of Pancreas, a progressive and categorized as medically incurable disease. But for Devansh Agrawal, it took exactly 2 and a half month of meeting our Nutrition therapist Meena Gupta and following the recommended DIP Diet to reverse and cure the incurable.

100

Hepatomegaly & Liver Abscess

Medical history of the patient :

Narendra Agrawal, 60 years, from Howrah, contacted our Diabetes Educator & Nutrition Therapist Meena Gupta on 4 April 2020

Diagnosis: Liver Abscess, hepatomegaly, BP from 30yrs, gall bladder sludge, polycystic kidney disease

Discomforts: Consistent 103^0 Fever even after consuming antibiotics for 15 days, Severe Pain, Indigestion, Vomiting, Swelling in the Legs.

Medicine/Intervention: Gozee 500, Trozte-D, Ravitoo, Lycoxy, Metroyl

Intervention (Diet Therapy): The customized DIP diet plan was followed from 6 April 2020 to be followed for 6 months

Outcome: After 2 months

Status: Liver abscess cured, hepatomegaly reduced in size

Discomforts: Nil

Medications: Nil

Life -saving W.I.S.E truth:

At the age of 60 years, with a collection of life-threatening diseases, affecting at least four major organs (liver, kidney, heart and gallbladder) and a handful of medicines, life is expected to become worsewith every passing day. But for Narendra Agrawal, it was a pleasant U-turn, ever since he met our Nutrition Therapist Meena Gupta and started following the DIP Diet. Now at the time of publication of the book, he is leading a healthy life with zero medication and zero discomfort.

101

Migraine & Diabetes

Medical history of the patient:

Varun Bhargav, 52 years, from New Delhi, India contacted our Diabetes Educator Vishal Saini in 2018

Diagnosis: Migraine, Diabetes,

Discomforts: High blood sugar readings, frequent migraine, Acidity

Medicine/ medical intervention: 80 units of Insulin/ day

Intervention (Diet Therapy): The customized DIP diet plan was followed for 3 months in 2018 and subsequently followed standard DIP Diet till now.

Outcome: In just 40 days

Status: Insulin units reduced from 80 units to 17 units per day, No more migraine, no more acidity, 6 kg weight loss

Discomforts: Nil

Medications: Now Taking 17 units of Insulin per day.

Life -saving W.I.S.E truth:

Migraine, for majority of the patients, is understood as a lifelong suffering but not for Varun, specially after he met our Diabetes educator Vishal Saini. He lost a lot in the 1st 40 days of adopting the DIP Diet and also lost 6 kg of weight. He also lost majority of insulin dependency, no more acidity and, of course, no more migraine.

102

Metabolic Syndrome

Medical history of the patient at the time when he contacted us:

Sandeep Trehan, 53years, from New Delhi, India contacted us on 7 December 2020 through W.I.S.E and assigned to W.I.S.E Expert Hema Singh.

Diagnosis: Diabetes Type 2, High BP, High Cholesterol

Discomforts: Mouth Blisters, high sugar readings, High blood pressure

Medicine/medical intervention: Trajenta Duo, Ecosprin, Prolomet

Intervention (Diet Therapy): The customized '3 Weeks' W.I.S.E protocol' was followed from 8 December 2020 and subsequently followed standard DIP Diet

Outcome: After 3 weeks

Present Status: Sugar and BP readings in healthy range, cholesterol levels normal

Discomforts: Nil

Medications: Nil

Life -saving W.I.S.E truth:

At the time of contacting our W.I.S.E service, Sandeep Trehan was a classic case of metabolic syndrome i.e., a combination of three medical conditions Diabetes, High BP and High Cholesterol. Immediately after following DIP Diet, he not only got rid of all the medicines but completely overcame his so-called metabolic syndrome.

SECTION -IV

Clinical trial of the DIP Diet

by

All India Institute of Ayurveda

(Under Ministry of AYUSH,

Govt. of India)

Ctri/2018/12/016654

The Final Words

To see the effectiveness of the DIP Diet, clinical trial was conducted by All India Institute of Ayurveda, under the CTRI number CTRI/2018/12/016654.

The last two lines of the above trial (as published in www.ctri.nic.in) summarizes perfectly about the usefulness of DIP Diet in the prevention and cure of the disease.

The last two lines of the trial are as follows:

> *'Just by the administration of proper food and diet it is possible to cure the diseases even without the need of administration of medicines and treatment.(ka.sm.khl.4/5) Any disease can be comprehensively cured without any medicine by just following 'pathya Ahara' or wholesome food whereas even hundreds of medicines and formulations cannot cure a disease in the absence of a planned wholesome regimen of diet.'*

FULL DETAILS (Read-only) -> Click Here to Create PDF for Current Dataset of Trial

CTRI Number	**CTRI/2018/12/016654** [Registered on: 13/12/2018] **Trial Registered Prospectively**
Last Modified On:	12/12/2018
Post Graduate Thesis	Yes
Type of Trial	Interventional
Type of Study	Medical Device Ayurveda
Study Design	Other
Public Title of Study	Role of agnikarma and diet in lower back pain
Scientific Title of Study	A CLINICAL STUDY ON AGNIKARMA AND DIP(DISCIPLINED AND INTELLIGENT PERSON)DIET IN THE MANAGEMENT OF KATIGATASANDHI VATA WITH SPECIAL REFERENCE TO LUMBAR SPONDYLOSIS.
Trial Acronym	
Secondary IDs if Any	**Secondary ID**: NIL; **Identifier**: NIL

Secondary IDs if Any

Secondary ID	Identifier
NIL	NIL

Details of Principal Investigator or overall Trial Coordinator (multi-center study)

Name	DR S K GUPTA
Designation	H.O.D Dept. OF SHALYA TANTRA
Affiliation	All india institute of ayurveda,mathura road,gautampuri,sarita vihar,new delhi-76
Address	Department of shalya Tantra 5th floor academic block,All india institute of ayurveda,sarita vihar, gautampuri, new delhi South DELHI 110076 India
Phone	8368403099
Fax	
Email	drskgupta17@gmail.com

Details of Contact Person Scientific Query

Name	DR S K GUPTA
Designation	H.O.D Dept. OF SHALYA TANTRA
Affiliation	All india institute of ayurveda,mathura road,gautampuri,sarita vihar,new delhi-76
Address	Department of shalya Tantra 5th floor academic block,All india institute of ayurveda,sarita vihar, gautampuri, new delhi South West DELHI 110076 India
Phone	8368403099
Fax	

	Email: drskgupta17@gmail.com
Details of Contact Person Public Query	**Name**: DrMONIKA SODE **Designation**: PG Scholar 1st year **Affiliation**: All india institute of ayurveda,mathura road,gautampuri,sarita vihar,new delhi-76 **Address**: Department of shalya Tantra 5th floor academic block,All india institute of ayurveda,sarita vihar, gautampuri, new delhi South DELHI 110076 India **Phone**: 9540596304 **Fax**: **Email**: monikasode0@gmail.com
Source of Monetary or Material Support	All India Institute of Ayurveda, New Delhi
Primary Sponsor	**Name**: all india institute of ayurveda **Address**: All India Institute of Ayurveda, Matura Road,Gautam puri,Sarita Vihar **Type of Sponsor**: Research institution and hospital
Details of Secondary Sponsor	**Name**: NIL **Address**: NIL
Countries of Recruitment	India

Sites of Study — No of Sites = **1**

Name of Principal Investigator	Name of Site	Site Address	Phone/Fax/Email
Dr Monika Sode	All India Institute of Ayurveda	OPD No 6, Ground Floor, Hospital Block, South West DELHI	9540596304 monikasode0@gmail.com

Details of Ethics Committee — No of Ethics Committees= **1**

Name of Committee	Approval Status
IEC	Approved

Regulatory Clearance Status from DCGI	**Status** Not Applicable
Health Condition / Problems Studied	**Health Type**: Patients **Condition**: **(1) ICD-10 Condition:** M478||Other spondylosis,
Intervention / Comparator Agent	see table below
Inclusion Criteria	see table below
ExclusionCriteria	**Details**: Patients of DM, TB of spine, fracture of spine, HIV, HBsAG, VDRL, osteopenia / osteoporosis or fracture of lumbar spine, Spondylolisthesis, ankylosing spondylosis, rheumatoid arthritis, Malignancy of lumbar vertebra
Method of Generating Random Sequence	Computer generated randomization
Method of Concealment	An Open list of random numbers
Blinding/Masking	Open Label
Primary Outcome	see table below
Secondary Outcome	see table below
Target Sample Size	**Total Sample Size="90"** **Sample Size from India="90"** **Final Enrollment numbers achieved (Total)=** "Applicable only for Completed/Terminated trials" **Final Enrollment numbers achieved (India)=**"Applicable only for Completed/Terminated trials"

Intervention / Comparator Agent

Type	Name	Details
Comparator Agent	Agni Karma	Four sessions of Agnikarma with Bindu dahan vishesha by pancha dhatushalaka at the interval of 7 days.
Intervention	Agni Karma with DIP Diet	Four sessions of Agnikarma with Bindu dahan vishesha by pancha dhatushalaka at the interval of 7 days. This will be associated with DIP DIET - Daily for 1 month

Inclusion Criteria

Age From	20.00 Year(s)
Age To	60.00 Year(s)
Gender	Both
Details	Patients irrespective to their sex, religion, education and socio-economic status with cardinal features of Lumbar Spondylosis.

Primary Outcome

Outcome	TimePoints
Relief in cardinal symptoms of lumbar spondylosis.	One Month

Secondary Outcome

Outcome	TimePoints
Improvement in quality of life by WHO QOL Scale.	18 months

Phase of Trial	Phase 2/ Phase 3
Date of First Enrollment (India)	20/12/2018
Date of Study Completion (India)	Applicable only for Completed/Terminated trials
Date of First Enrollment (Global)	Date Missing
Date of Study Completion (Global)	Applicable only for Completed/Terminated trials
Estimated Duration of Trial	**Years="1"** **Months="6"** **Days="0"**
Recruitment Status of Trial (Global)	Not Applicable
Recruitment Status of Trial (India)	Not Yet Recruiting
Publication Details	THE thesis work will be publish in reputed journal
Individual Participant Data (IPD) Sharing Statement	**Will individual participant data (IPD) be shared publicly (including data dictionaries)?**
Brief Summary	Sandhigata Vata is a clinical condition develops when vitiated Vayuis localized at Kati Pradesha.The symptoms likeShoola, Shopha, Stambha etc. are developed.During the process of pathogenesis, Kapha Avrit VyanVayu obstruct the circulation of Rasa RaktaDhatu and gradually structural changes are developed in Kati Pardesha.Acharya Charak has described this disease first time as'Sandhigata Anila' under the chapter of Vatavyadhi(ch.ch.28/36). It is characterized by the features of Shoola (pain),Shotha (swelling) and Akunchana Prasarane Vedana (pain on flexion and extension of the joint), Hantisandhin (structural changes). Madhava has given one extra feature i.e. Aatopa (crepitus). Based upon its feature,Sandhigata Vata can be equated withLumbar Spondylosis. Lumbar Spondylosis is a degenerative condition which affects the lower spine. In a patient with Lumbar Spondylosis, the spine is compromised by a narrowing of the space between the vertebrae, causing a variety of health problems ranging from back pain to neurological issues. WHO estimates that about 80% of individuals older than 40 years have lumbar spondylosis, increasing from 3% of individuals aged 20-29 years. Internationally, lumbar spondylosis can be developed in persons as young as 20 years. It increases with, and perhaps is an inevitable concomitant of age.Inmodern medicine various treatment options are available like conservative treatment, surgical methods but all modalities have their own limitation and complications. In Ayurveda Snehana, Upanaha, Agnikarma, Raktamokshana, Katibasti, Virechana, Bhesaja Chikitsa etc. have been recommended for management of Vatikdisorders. Among these Agnikarma is a well-known para-surgical procedure and has its own therapeutic value for treatment of Sandhigata Vata(Lumbar spondylosis). Acharya Sushruta has mentioned Agnikarmaprocedure as a best among all otherprocedure(su.su 12/3)and in this study Pancha Dhatu Shalaka has been

selected for Agnikarma. It is suitable for heat transfer and to produce Samyak Dagdha Vrana (ideal therapeutic burn). पथ्येऽसतिगदातस्यतिमऔषधतिषेवर्त: ।। पथ्येसतिगदातस्यतिमऔषधतिषेवर्त: ।। (लोतलम्बराज) That means those people have no use to givemedicine who did not follow proper diet. And for those who actually follow proper diet there is no need of medicine for them. Ahara(food), Nidra (sleep) and Brahmacharya (celibacy) are the Traya Upastambhas (Trayopastambhas) explained in Ayurveda. Among the three pillars, Ahara or food is a major supporting pillar which helps in sustenance of life and maintenance of health. One cannot imagine living without food. Acharya Charaka Samhita gives a beautiful concept about Ahara and tells that the Ahara not only forms this body but also forms the diseases which occur in us. If the wholesome food (Hita Ahara) is responsible for Sukha (happiness, health), the unwholesome food (AhitaAhara) causes Dukha (misery, unhealthy). He also tells that Ahara or food is the best among the things which sustain the life.(ch.su.28/45) Kashyapa tells that no medicine is equivalent to the Aharaor food. He also calls Ahara as Maha Bhaishajya (greatest and best medicine). Just by the administration of proper food and diet it is possible to cure the diseases even without the need of administration of medicines and treatment.(ka.sm.khl.4/5) Any disease can be comprehensively cured without any medicine by just following 'pathya Ahara' or wholesome food whereas even hundreds of medicines and formulations cannot cure a disease in the absence of a planned wholesome regimen of diet.

Close

Conclusion:

Lumbar Spondylosis due to its clinical manifestation, pathogenesis and complication can be positively correlated with Katishoola. Etiological factors mentioned under common Vata Prakopa stand true as etiological factors for Lumbar Spondylosis.

- In present study majority of the patients had Dwandwaj Prakruti i.e. Vatakapha or Vata-pittaj. Also majority of patients had Vishamagni and Krura Koshtha. All these finding support the dominance of Vata Dosha.
- Combination in group-B is more potent in mitigating Vata and Kapha and also gives nutrition to the body which gives a good impact of bone health.
- Nitric Oxide required opening the hidden arteries at the moment of emergency and the only way to help body enhance the production of nitric oxide by eating more than 50% of your diet as DIP Diet.
- Importance of diet should be understand by everyone because whole body metabolism depends on the food what we eat that should be plant based.
- Eating a DIP Diet actually have a significantly lower risk of bone disorder even though they may be consuming less calcium because people who eat a lot of meat and dairy product, they excreate more calcium,so the net effect is to leach calcium from their bone.

- Atherosclerosis can obstruct the arteries that feed the spine, and diminish blood flow resulting in disc degeneration causing LS.
- Any intervention reversing atherosclerosis will have the potential to halt and even reverse LS.
- Diet rich in fruits and raw vegetables with zero animal food/diary product (as in DIP Diet) has proven to reverse atherosclerosis.
- Nitric Oxide required to open the hidden arteries at the moment of emergency and the only way to help body enhance the production of nitric oxide by eating more than 50% of your diet as DIP Diet.
- Preventive aspect and patient's education play an important role in the management of Katishoola.
- Proper guidelines about posture etc along with exercise strengthening the spine are helpul for effective management.

Thus null hypothesis is rejected and alternate hypothesis is accepted i.e. The application of 4 sessions of Agnikarma with Bindu Dahan Veshesa by Pancha Dhatu Shalaka at the interval of 7days and 4 sessions of Agnikarma with Bindu Dahan Veshesa by Pancha Dhatu Shalaka at the interval of 7days along with DIP Diet for one 1month is found effective in the management of KatiSandhigata Vata (lumbar spondylosis).

SECTION -V

Joint Statement on Safety and Efficacy of COVID-19 Vaccine

(Signed by 111 Doctors from across the country)

Joint Statement on Safety and Efficacy of COVID-19 Vaccine (Signed by 111 Doctors from across the country)

The very understanding of the microbe and its role in human sickness (by the mainstream medical system) should be questioned in general and specifically in case of COVID-19, as we now know that according to CDC-USA, people who wore masks suffered from COVID-19 20 times (2000%) more than the people who did not wear a mask. Further, the fatality rate of just 0.1% in COVID-19 (comparable to Flu) does not warrant any special precaution including vaccination.

Q1. Does the vaccine qualify the "Gold standard" of epidemiologic studies, the Randomized Double Blind Placebo Control (RDBPC) Studies?

Answer: As of now it is safe to believe that no Randomized Double Blind Placebo Control (RDBPC) studies have taken place till they are published in peer reviewed medical journal.

Q2. In India, Astra Zeneca got approval to launch COVID-19 vaccine (Covishield). Can we rely on the data about the safety of vaccines provided by Astra Zeneca?

Answer: In the past, Astra Zeneca has been guilty of giving wrong data at least 12 times, amounting to a penalty of about $617241159 which is equal to INR 45,05,86,04,607 (Forty-five hundred crore, eighty-six lakh, four thousand six hundred seven rupees).

The above data shows that the efficacy and safety of Astra Zeneca vaccine cannot be trusted.

Q3. Can we rule out the long-term side effects of COVID-19 vaccine such as Infertility, Paralysis, Neurological disorder and death?

Answer: The vaccine has not been tested for its long-term effects so the above side effects cannot be ruled out.

Q4. As the vaccination drive has already started in the US and the UK, what is the rate of side effects?

Answer: As on December 18, 2020, CDC - USA reported that out of 1,12807 vaccinated participants, 3,150 participants would not be able to perform normal daily activities and would require care from the doctor.

Q5. Is the COVID-19 vaccine safe for people allergic to any food/ medicine etc.?

Answer: COVID-19 vaccine is known to cause allergic reactions in certain people and may even cause Paralysis and death. The Government of UK has recommended avoiding the vaccine if you are allergic to any type of food or medicine. Remember each of us can be allergic to some medicine or food.

Q6. For how long will the vaccine be effective?

Answer: Based on the present evidences, the best estimate for the effectiveness of vaccine is maximum two months.

Q7. Since the animal product (Fetal Bovine Serum- FBS) is used in the COVID-19 vaccine, has any technology or screening method been used to rule out the accidental jump of new virus from animals to humans through this vaccine?

Answer: Presently, there is no fool proof screening method available (with the science) to exclude any previously unknown virus from entering into the new vaccine.

Only when millions of people take the vaccine and remain healthy (without having any unexpected adverse reaction) for about 5 years, it will be safe to assume that the vaccine is free of any unknown/new virus.

Q8. In India, if a person gets adverse life-threatening side effects due to COVID 19 vaccine, is there any compensation from the Vaccine Company or the Government of India?

Answer: In UK, about an equivalent of INR 1,20,000,00 is given to the patients injured through the vaccine. In USA also, there is Vaccine Adverse Event Reporting System (VAERS) through which vaccine injured patients are compensated. In 2020, an equivalent of about INR 2000 crore was distributed to vaccine injured people. In India, however there is no such provision, which means Indians can go ahead vaccinating themselves at their own risk.

Q9. Will this COVID-19 vaccine protect against the new variant of SARS-CoV-2?

Answer: There is no evidence to prove the efficacy of COVID-19 vaccine on the new variant SARS-CoV-2. Till then, it is safe to assume that COVID-19 vaccine will not protect against the new SARS-CoV-2 variant/strain.

Q10. Will I be free of the mask and social distancing guidelines, once I vaccinate myself with COVID-19 vaccine?

Answer: No, vaccinating is like voluntarily infecting yourself with the SARS-CoV-2 virus with the hope that it will help the body to produce antibodies against it.

In fact, all vaccinated persons should quarantine themselves for 14 days in the same way as when someone catches infection naturally.

Date: 6th January, 2021

Convener

- Dr Amar Singh Azad
  MD (Paediatrics), MD (Community Medicine)

Co-Conveners

- Dr Biswaroop Roy Chowdhury *(Ph. D Diabetes),*
- Dr K. B. Tumane *(Chest Specialist-MBBS),*
- Ex-IAS Dr Praveen Kumar *(Senior Homeopath)*

Signatories

- Dr Nilesh Chintamani Patil (MBBS, Orthopaedic Surgeon)
- Dr Satish Malhotra (MBBS, MD)
- Dr Sandeep Sharma (MBBS)
- Dr Mathew Anthony Puthuparampil (MD)
- Dr B N Pandey (MBBS, MD)
- Dr Lovleen (MBBS, MD)
- Dr Pallavi Nilesh Patil (MBBS, DMRE)
- Dr Arvind Bhardwaj (MBBS, PGDMCH)
- Dr Rajani Engu (MBBS, MD)
- Dr Seema Arora (MBBS)
- Dr S. Sunitha (MBBS DMRD Radiologist)
- Dr Shyam Sunder Gupta (MBBS, MD)
- Dr Archana Satyam (MBBS)
- Dr Nisha Chidrawar (MBBS)

- Dr Madhab Nayak (MBBS, MD)
- Dr Rajratna Ingle (MBBS, MD)
- Dr Harini R Jakkipally (MBBS, MD)
- Dr Manisha Chandel (MBBS, MD)
- Dr Sorubini Loganathan (MBBS, MD)
- Dr Harish Sharma (BAMS, MD)
- Dr Rahul Kumar Vaidhya (BAMS)
- Dr Mahendra Kosariya (BAMS)
- Dr Pradip Mahadev Kelkar (BAMS)
- Dr Navneet Kaur (BAMS)
- Dr Pankaj Patidar (BAMS, CRAV)
- Dr Manoj Warware (BHMS)
- Dr Amarjit Singh Mann (BHMS)
- Dr Shyam Narayan Pandey (M Sc, Ph D (Geriatric Care), ND, FCNR)
- Dr Indupreet Kaur (BDS)
- Dr Dharmesh Thakkar (BDS)
- Dr Sanju Khari (BDS)
- Dr Swati Sharma (BDS)
- Anamika Singh (BPT)
- Dr Jasvir Kaur (DHMS)
- Dr Ashok Singhal (BAMS, MD)
- Dr Brij Bhushan Goel (Naturopath)
- Dr Ajay Tiwari (Homeopath)
- Dr Sudhakar (Ad. D.Acu., BEMS, MD. (EH) NDDY)
- Dr Jacob Vadakkanchery (DNYS, Honorary Professor, Shobith University)
- Dr Atul Ramesh Narkhede (BHMS)
- Dr Pankaj Chaudhary (BHMS)
- Dr Nidhi Jain (BHMS)
- Dr Manoj Kumar Sharma (BHMS)
- Dr Shaikh Iqra Ayaz (BAMS)
- Dr Shaikh Warisha Nasim (BUMS)
- Dr Vishal Singh Chauhan (BHMS, M.D)

- Dr Abhishek Singh (BHMS)
- Dr Azheruddin (BUMS)
- Dr Goutam Paul (DBMS)
- Dr Raj Bhagat (BDS, PGDCC)
- Dr Shivam Bathri (BAMS)
- Dr Rashmi M Patil (BAMS)
- Dr Lokesh Joshi (BAMS)
- Dr Pardeep kumar dhiman (BHMS)
- Dr Hemshanakar Sahu (BHMS)
- Dr Karanraj Sandip Deshmukh (BHMS)
- Dr Anu Shreeya Das (BAMS)
- Dr Rajeev chaubey (BHMS)
- Dr Ranjeet satre (BHMS)
- Dr Rajeev kumar (BDS)
- Dr Prashant Sharma (BAMS, MD)
- Dr Hafsa (BUMS)
- Dr Bhupendra Ghadia (DHMS)
- Dr Nikhil Khairnar (BAMS)
- Dr Prakash Singh (BAMS)
- Dr Ashok Kumar Chinni (BDS)
- Dr Geet Priya (BDS)
- Dr Satish (BDS)
- Dr Avtar Singh Vilkhu (DHMS)
- Dr Bhupinder Singh (DHMS)
- Dr Chander Kant (BHMS)
- Dr Jaswinder Kaur Sethi (BHMS)
- Dr Kunwar Aryaman (BHMS)
- Dr Anupama K M (BAMS)
- Dr Pankaj Sital (BAMS)
- Dr Harsha Bhorahari (BAMS)
- Dr Sanjay Kumar Patel (BHMS)
- Dr Lakshminarayan Reddy (BAMS)
- Dr Yuditya Godara (MAMS)

- Dr Arvind Katiyar (MHMS)
- Dr Honey Godara (BHMS)
- Dr Deepak Prabhakar Mishra (BAMS)
- Dr Ameet Shimpi (BAMS)
- Dr Bhavik Ghanshyambhai Rana (BHMS)
- Dr Vishal Singh Chauhan (BHMS)
- Dr Atul Kumar (BAMS)
- Dr Mehul Rajgor (BAMS)
- Dr Indu (BHMS)
- Dr Kishan Kumar (BAMS)
- Dr Lathiya Dharaben Himmatbhai (BHMS)
- Dr Praveen G Pateliya (BHMS)
- Dr Ramya PR (BHMS)
- Dr Surekha Singh (BAMS)
- Dr Sahid Akhter (BAMS)
- Dr Akshata K Alagundagi (BAMS)
- Dr Jitendra Singh (BAMS)
- Dr Himmat (BHMS)
- Dr Veena P Kumbar (BAMS)
- Dr Rohan Dumbre (BAMS)
- Dr Neelam Thakur (BAMS)
- Dr Milan Biswas (BAMS)
- Dr Manoj Kumar (BAMS)
- Dr J Preet Anand (BAMS)
- Dr Sangram Bavachakar (BAMS)
- Dr Mehershobha P Vyas (BHMS)
- Dr Brajendra Yadav (BHMS)
- Dr Hemlata Gupta (BHMS)

Let every morning be the Hunza Morning

If you have decided to pick only one of my suggestions for the sake of your health, then take this suggestion :

Stop consuming tea specially, morning tea. The early morning tea makes the inner lining of your intestinal wall acidic, as after a long night of fasting your stomach is empty and craving for food. An acidic stomach on a regular basis is the single biggest cause of all kind of inflammatory and lifestyle diseases including arthritis, Diabetes etc.

How to stop craving of tea ⟶ Switch to Hunza Tea

Hunza Civilization: Hunza people are the Indians living at extreme northwest of India in Hindu Kush range. They are known to be one of the world's healthiest civilizations, often living up to the age of 110 years.

How to prepare Hunza Tea (serves four):

Ingredients:

- 12 Mint leaves(Pudina)
- 8 Basil Leaves(Tulsi)
- 4 Green cardamom (Elaichi)
- 2 gm Cinnamon (Dalchini)
- 20 gm Ginger (Adrak)
- 20 gm Jaggery (Gur)

Instructions:

- Take 4 cups of water in a tea pan
- Add all ingredients, simmer it for 10mins
- Add a dash of lemon juice and serve hot or cold